Clinical Seizure Semiology: Localization, Lateralization, and Network Interpretation

A structured review organized by lobe and sublobar localization, with a practical methodology for semiologic sequence analysis

Prepared for clinical and presurgical epilepsy interpretation

Author: Rene Andrade Machado

Associate professor of neurology

Nemours Children's Hospital, Orlando

To the patient who suffer from epilepsy

"It appears to me to be no more divine nor more sacred than other diseases, but has a natural cause … like other affections. Men regard its nature and cause as divine from ignorance".

Hippocrates

Contents

How to Use This Book

This guide helps readers enter the monograph efficiently while preserving the sequence-first method that anchors the rest of the text.

- Read Chapter 1 first if you want a shared method for reconstructing onset, spread, and postictal interpretation.
- Read Chapters 10 to 12 early if you need the highest-yield bedside lateralizers, common diagnostic traps, and safeguards against overinterpretation.
- Use Appendix A during video review, Appendix H for structured questioning, and Appendix F when you need an explicit confidence statement.
- Use Appendices B, G, and I as quick-reference tools during conference, and use Appendices C and J when you want the underlying evidence base.

Throughout the book, give the earliest symptom or first objective sign more weight than later propagated features.

Abstract

Seizure semiology remains one of the most clinically useful, immediately available, and cost-effective tools for inferring the seizure onset zone and the side of onset in focal epilepsy, especially when interpreted in sequence rather than as isolated signs. The literature consistently shows that the best localizing information usually comes from the first subjective symptom or the earliest observable sign, whereas later manifestations increasingly reflect propagation through distributed cortical and subcortical networks. Across different reviewed articles, some patterns are particularly robust: unilateral clonic activity, unilateral tonic or dystonic posturing, and early versive head and eye deviation usually lateralize contralaterally; a figure-of-four posture lateralizes contralateral to the extended arm; the last clonic jerk of a bilateral tonic-clonic seizure tends to be ipsilateral to seizure onset; hemifield visual aura usually lateralizes to the contralateral occipital lobe; and preserved awareness during temporal automatisms points toward the non-dominant hemisphere. At the same time, the papers repeatedly emphasize the limitations of semiology: inter-rater variability, overlap among lobes, rapid spread from deep or mesial sources, and the fact that symptomatogenic cortex may lie outside the true seizure-onset zone. This review therefore begins with a methodology for practical semiologic analysis, then proceeds by lobe and sublobar localization—frontal, temporal, insular/perisylvian, parietal, precuneal, occipital, anterior cingulate, posterior cingulate, and special network-related seizures—and ends with a detailed critique of the limitations of semiology-based localization and lateralization.

Executive clinical message

- Interpret seizures as dynamic sequences, not as static lists of signs.
- Weight the first aura or first objective sign more heavily than later signs.
- Use anatomo-clinical correlation to decide whether a sign is likely to reflect onset, early spread, or late network recruitment.
- Treat highly specific but poorly localizing signs differently from highly lateralizing but non-localizing signs.
- Never use semiology in isolation when scalp EEG, MRI, PET, invasive EEG, or neuropsychology are discordant.

Introduction

Why semiology still matters

Seizure semiology remains one of the most immediately available, clinically grounded, and cost-effective tools for the evaluation of focal epilepsy. Despite major advances in structural and functional neuroimaging, molecular genetics, and invasive electrophysiology, the careful observation and interpretation of ictal symptoms and signs continue to play a central role in localizing and lateralizing seizure onset, guiding diagnostic hypotheses, and informing presurgical planning. Semiology is present at the bedside, available before any test is ordered, and uniquely reflects the patient's lived experience of the seizure. Yet, as consistently emphasized across the modern epilepsy literature, seizure semiology is also one of the most frequently misunderstood and overinterpreted domains in clinical practice.

Why sequence matters more than sign lists

This book is built on a central premise supported by decades of clinical observation and validated by intracranial EEG studies: seizures must be interpreted as **dynamic sequences**, not as static collections of signs. The earliest subjective symptom or the first unequivocal objective sign usually carries the highest localizing and lateralizing value, whereas later manifestations increasingly reflect propagation through anatomically distributed cortical and subcortical networks. A seizure that ends as bilateral asymmetric tonic posturing, hypermotor behavior, or secondary generalization does not necessarily begin in the frontal lobe; rather, its final appearance may be the consequence of rapid recruitment of motor systems from a posterior, temporal, insular, or cingulate onset. The discipline of semiologic interpretation therefore lies not in memorizing associations between signs and lobes, but in reconstructing seizure chronology and assigning appropriate anatomical weight to each phase of the event.

Core anatomo-clinical framework

At the core of this approach is the distinction among the **symptomatogenic zone**, the **seizure onset zone**, and the **epileptogenic zone**. The symptomatogenic zone refers to the cortical region whose activation produces a particular symptom or sign; it may lie adjacent to, overlap with, or be remote from the true seizure onset zone. The epileptogenic zone, in turn, represents the minimum cortical territory that must be treated or disconnected to achieve seizure freedom. These zones frequently overlap in mesial temporal epilepsy and primary motor cortex epilepsy, but they diverge substantially in parietal, insular, orbitofrontal, cingulate, and network-driven epilepsies. Failure to honor these distinctions is a major source of mislocalization, particularly when prominent propagated motor or autonomic features dominate the bedside impression.

This volume synthesizes an extensive contemporary and classic evidence base—including broad practical reviews, systematic analyses, intracranial EEG series, and focused cohort studies—to provide a disciplined, lobe-by-lobe and sublobar framework for semiologic interpretation. Rather than presenting semiology as a checklist of signs, the text emphasizes **temporal weighting**, **anatomical plausibility**, and **propagation pathways**. The earliest symptom is treated as the strongest clinical approximation of symptomatogenic cortex. Later signs are interpreted in light of known connectivity patterns, explaining why the same seizure can appear temporal, frontal, or generalized depending on when the observer begins to watch.

A recurring theme throughout the book is that some signs are highly **lateralizing** but poorly **localizing**, while others are anatomically specific but weak for hemispheric side. Early true versive head and eye deviation, unilateral dystonia, unilateral tonic or clonic motor activity, fencing posture, figure-of-four, the last clonic jerk of a generalized convulsion, Todd paresis, and postictal aphasia are among the most reliable lateralizing signs in focal epilepsy. In contrast, elementary sensory, auditory, visual, and vestibular auras can be remarkably localizing when carefully characterized, yet may offer only limited side certainty. Confident interpretation requires recognizing what a sign can and cannot tell us, and resisting the temptation to overextend its significance beyond its validated scope.

How this book is organized

The book is organized anatomically, progressing from frontal lobe epilepsy through temporal, insular, parietal, occipital, precuneal, and cingulate epilepsies, before addressing special seizure networks and high-yield lateralizing signs. Frontal lobe epilepsy is approached as a spectrum of motor and premotor syndromes shaped by rapid propagation and network recruitment. Primary motor cortex seizures present with the clearest pathophysiologic semiology, including contralateral focal clonic activity and Jacksonian march. Supplementary motor area epilepsy is characterized by abrupt, often sleep-related seizures featuring asymmetric bilateral tonic posturing, while frontal eye field recruitment produces early forced version. Orbitofrontal and anterior cingulate seizures illustrate how deeply situated cortex can generate prominent behavioral, emotional, and autonomic manifestations despite limited scalp EEG expression.

Temporal lobe epilepsy, the most extensively studied focal epilepsy, is presented with explicit differentiation among mesial, lateral neocortical, temporal pole, and temporal-plus patterns. The primacy of the aura—particularly epigastric rising, experiential phenomena, simple auditory symptoms, vertigo, and visual disturbances—is emphasized over later automotor behavior. The text highlights classic lateralizing features such as unilateral dystonia, preserved awareness during automatisms in non-dominant temporal epilepsy, and language disturbances pointing to hemisphere dominance. Importantly, temporal-plus epilepsy is treated not as an academic curiosity, but as a practical explanation for surgical failures and discordant presurgical data when posterior or extratemporal onset is overlooked.

Insular epilepsy is framed as one of the most deceptive focal epilepsies due to its deep location and extensive connectivity. Anterior insular seizures produce complex viscerosensory and autonomic symptoms, often including laryngeal constriction, hypersalivation, nausea, and diffuse bodily discomfort, while posterior insular seizures more frequently generate painful, burning, or dysesthetic sensory experiences. Throughout this section, the emphasis is on pattern recognition rather than single-sign localization, and on understanding how insular seizures rapidly assume temporal or frontal characteristics.

Parietal lobe epilepsy receives particular attention because of its extraordinary semiologic diversity and its frequent misclassification. The text underscores the importance of subjective phenomena—somatosensory aura, sensory march, pain, body schema distortion, kinetopsia, vestibular illusions, and altered self-perception—as primary localizing clues. Medial parietal seizures arising from the precuneus are highlighted for their characteristic vestibular and perceptual onset with rapid frontal propagation, a pattern that often leads to false frontal localization if the early symptoms are ignored.

Occipital lobe epilepsy is presented with careful differentiation between elementary visual aura arising from primary visual cortex and complex visual phenomena associated with visual association areas and parieto-occipital networks. The practical distinction between epileptic visual aura and migraine aura is emphasized, along with the lateralizing value of hemifield visual symptoms and ocular signs such as epileptic nystagmus and unilateral blinking.

The cingulate cortex is treated as a network rather than a single entity. Anterior cingulate epilepsy is characterized by affective-autonomic and hypermotor syndromes, often including fear, screaming, and vocalization, whereas posterior cingulate epilepsy—particularly ventral posterior cingulate and retrosplenial cortex involvement—frequently mimics temporal lobe epilepsy through rapid temporal propagation. The cingulate sections illustrate one of the book's key messages: some epilepsies can only be recognized by their propagation patterns and by the mismatch between bedside semiology and invasive anatomical truth.

Throughout the volume, limitations of semiology are addressed explicitly and repeatedly. Inter-rater variability, subjective recall, rapid propagation, deep or mesial sources, developmental effects in pediatric epilepsy, and the intrinsic difference between symptomatogenic and epileptogenic cortex all constrain what can be inferred from bedside observation alone. The book argues not for uncritical reliance on semiology, but for **disciplined integration** with scalp EEG, neuroimaging, functional imaging, invasive recordings, and neuropsychology. Discordance between modalities is treated as an analytic opportunity rather than an inconvenience.

Ultimately, this book advocates a shift in clinical habit: away from asking *"What lobe does this seizure look like?"* and toward asking *"What happened first, what happened next, and which parts of the sequence most plausibly reflect onset versus spread?"* By applying this sequence-based, anatomically grounded method, seizure semiology becomes not a relic of a pre-imaging era, but a sophisticated, indispensable tool for modern epilepsy practice—one that continues to shape diagnosis, surgical planning, and patient outcomes when used with appropriate rigor and humility.

CHAPTER 1

Methodology for Adequate Localization and Lateralization by Semiologic Sequence Analysis

The broad reviews converge on a core principle: the clinical value of semiology is maximal when the seizure is analyzed as a temporally ordered sequence. The first subjective symptom or the first reproducible objective sign is the best clinical approximation of symptomatogenic cortex, and therefore usually has the greatest localizing value. Later signs increasingly reflect spread, disinhibition, or network recruitment rather than true onset. Tufenkjian and Lüders explicitly propose that an ideal localizing sign should be easy to identify, reliable across observers, and among the earliest components of the seizure. Chowdhury and colleagues further emphasize that seizure manifestations evolve as the discharge propagates and that the symptomatogenic zone may lie close to, but not necessarily within, the epileptogenic zone (Tufenkjian & Lüders, 2012; Chowdhury et al., 2021).

The distinction among symptomatogenic zone, seizure onset zone, and epileptogenic zone is not semantic; it is the foundation of correct interpretation. The symptomatogenic zone is the cortical region whose activation or dysfunction produces a sign or symptom. The seizure onset zone is where clinical seizures actually start. The epileptogenic zone is the tissue that must be removed or disconnected to achieve seizure freedom. These zones often overlap, but the overlap is incomplete in many focal epilepsies, particularly in parietal, cingulate, insular, orbitofrontal, and network-rich epilepsies.

1.1 1.1 Conceptual framework

Concept	Practical meaning	Why it matters for semiology
Symptomatogenic zone	Region whose activation/dysfunction generates the observed symptom	The earliest aura or sign most often points here, not necessarily to the full epileptogenic region
Seizure onset zone (SOZ)	Region from which the seizure begins	Best estimated by integrating semiology with ictal EEG and imaging
Epileptogenic zone (EZ)	Region necessary for seizure generation and therefore the target of curative surgery	May be larger than the SOZ and may extend beyond symptomatogenic cortex

Concept	Practical meaning	Why it matters for semiology
Propagation pathway	Anatomical route by which the discharge reaches other cortical or subcortical areas	Explains why later signs can be misleading or falsely localizing
Lateralizing sign	Sign that indicates the side of onset but not the lobe or subregion	Examples include early version, unilateral dystonia, and postictal Todd paresis
Localizing sign	Sign that suggests a particular cortical region or lobe	Examples include elementary visual aura for primary visual cortex, auditory aura for Heschl gyrus, and marching sensory aura for primary sensory cortex

For day-to-day clinical work, the semiologic problem can be reframed as three sequential questions. First, what was the earliest symptom or sign? Second, what anatomical region would best explain that earliest event? Third, which later manifestations are more parsimoniously explained by spread? This disciplined approach is more useful than trying to map every feature directly onto a single cortical site.

1.2 Why timing matters

The practical guide by Chowdhury et al. explains that seizure propagation includes both a slow ictal wavefront and a much faster discharge spread. The slow wavefront reflects actual progressive recruitment of cortex and can explain phenomena such as Jacksonian march. The fast discharge can recruit connected regions quickly enough to produce semiology that appears nearly simultaneous from the bedside. This is one reason frontal and cingulate seizures can look explosive and why deep foci such as insula, orbitofrontal cortex, and posterior cingulate are frequently misidentified from surface appearances alone (Chowdhury et al., 2021).

Temporal weighting is therefore essential. In practice, semiologic data are best grouped into five windows: pre-ictal baseline context, first subjective symptom, first objective sign, evolving ictal pattern, and postictal state. The earliest two windows carry the strongest localizing power. The evolving ictal pattern is often useful for network inference. The postictal state frequently has lateralizing rather than localizing value.

Semiologic time window	Interpretive value	Typical examples	Caution
First subjective symptom	Highest localizing value when clear and reproducible	Epigastric rising, déjà vu, simple auditory aura, hemifield visual aura, unilateral distal paresthesia	Requires reliable recall and adequate awareness
First objective sign	Often highest combined localizing/lateralizing value	Contralateral clonus, fencing posture, early versive head turn, unilateral dystonia	Must distinguish true version from natural head movement
Early evolving pattern	Useful for onset-plus-early-spread inference	Automatisms after mesial temporal aura, tonic spread after sensory onset, behavioral arrest before hypermotor phase	Already partly contaminated by spread
Late ictal pattern	Usually better for network mapping than onset localization	Secondary generalization, bilateral tonic-clonic phase, hypermotor storm	Commonly misleading if over-weighted
Postictal state	Often lateralizing	Todd paresis, aphasia, nose wipe	Poor lobe localization in many cases

1.2 1.3 Stepwise practical workflow

1. Confirm that the spell is epileptic rather than dissociative, syncopal, or another nonepileptic paroxysmal event. In the uploaded review by Tufenkjian and Lüders, preserved awareness with eye flutter and the ability of bystanders to modify or alleviate the event favor dissociative seizures; alpha rhythm during apparent unresponsiveness is particularly persuasive against epilepsy.
2. Document the first subjective symptom word for word. The patient's original phenomenologic language should be preserved before the clinician translates it into semiologic categories.
3. Review video-EEG frame by frame and annotate the first unequivocal objective sign. Distinguish eye deviation from version, tonic stiffening from dystonia, and semipurposeful hypermotor behavior from automatisms.
4. Mark the latency of each major sign from electrographic or clinical onset. The same sign has different meaning depending on whether it occurs at 2 seconds, 20 seconds, or immediately before secondary generalization.
5. Build an anatomical hypothesis by matching earliest signs with known symptomatogenic cortex: for example, Heschl gyrus for simple auditory aura, primary visual cortex for elementary visual aura, postcentral gyrus for marching somatosensory aura, mesial temporal structures for epigastric rising plus experiential aura, and anterior insula for laryngeal constriction or visceral-autonomic onset.
6. Then explain later signs as spread. A parietal seizure that becomes tonic does not automatically become an SMA-onset seizure; the tonic component may simply indicate spread to mesial frontal motor networks.
7. Finally, reconcile the semiologic model with MRI, PET, scalp EEG, invasive EEG, and neuropsychology. Discordant semiology should trigger re-analysis, not forced agreement.

1.3 1.4 How to weight conflicting signs

A single seizure may contain both localizing and misleading elements. The practical rule is hierarchical weighting: earliest and anatomically specific signs outrank later and less specific signs. For example, a seizure beginning with unilateral distal contralateral paresthesia, then progressing to bilateral tonic posturing, should be interpreted first as postcentral or perirolandic/parietal rather than simply 'SMA' because the tonic phase can reflect spread. Similarly, a seizure with epigastric aura and déjà vu followed by automotor activity and late head version remains more consistent with mesial temporal onset than with frontal eye field onset, because the version is late.

When two robust lateralizing signs are concordant, confidence increases substantially. Tufenkjian and Lüders highlight that, in secondarily generalized seizures, a combination of version, tonic or clonic facial involvement, fencing posture, and figure-of-four can be stronger than any single sign considered in isolation.

Figure. Seizure with concordant early signs arising from the left hemisphere.

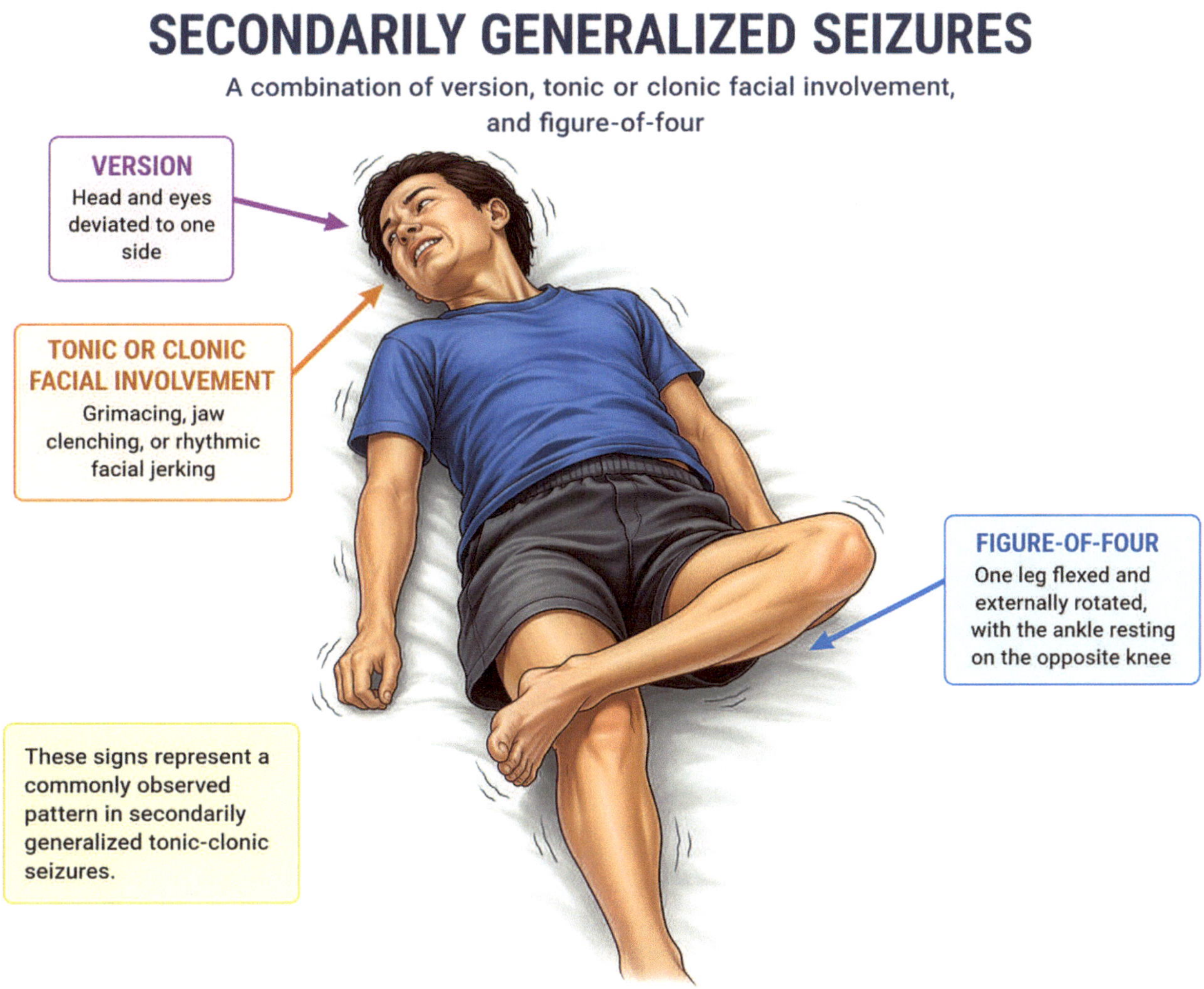

Figure 1. Conversely, when signs conflict—such as ipsilateral blinking but contralateral dystonia—priority should go to the earlier and better validated sign, while acknowledging uncertainty.

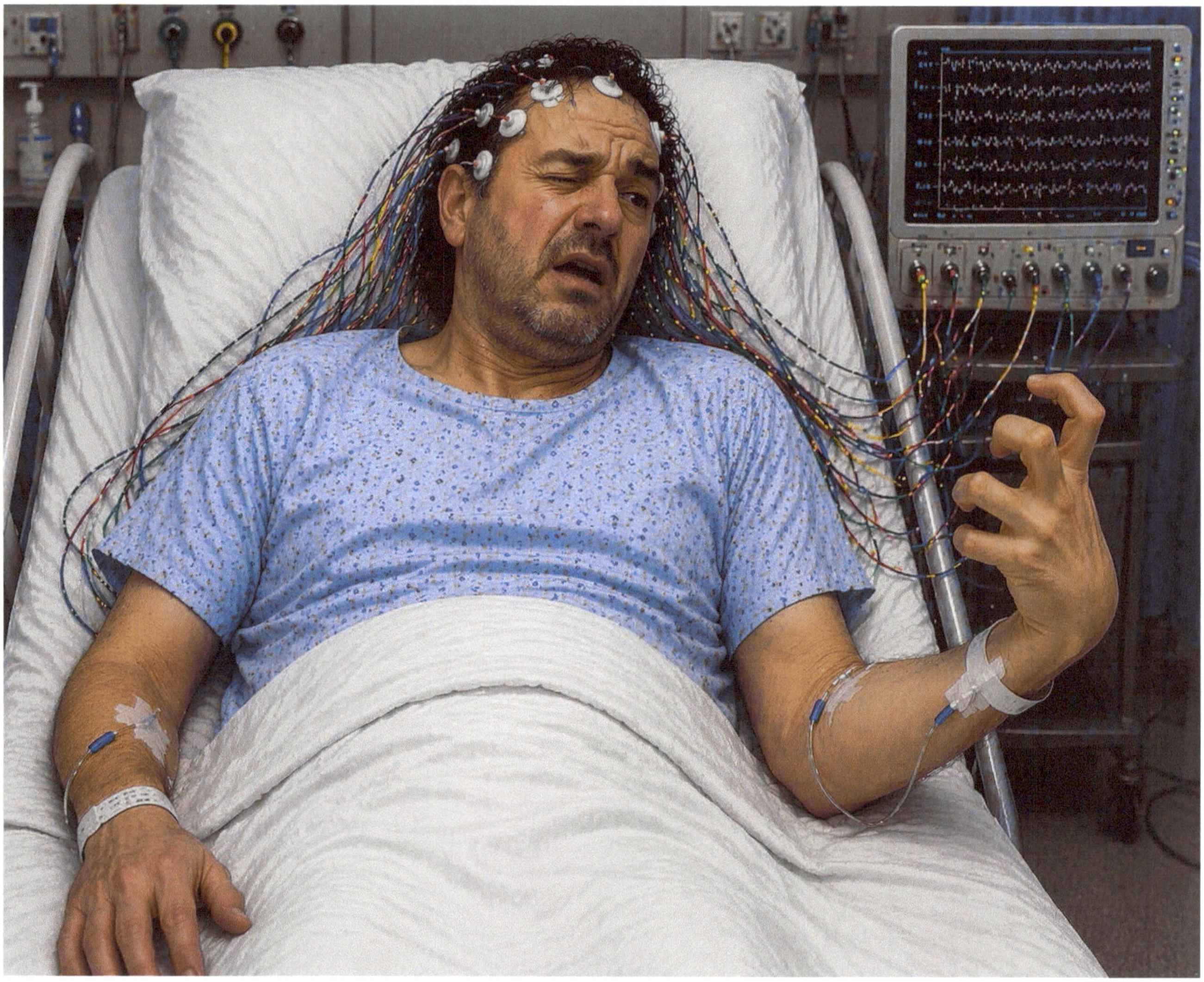

Figure 2. Conflicting signs in a patient with right temporal lobe epilepsy during the first 8 seconds of a typical seizure. Mild head deviation to the left is usually a left lateralizer, whereas left-hand ictal dystonia points contralaterally to right-sided onset. In this sequence, dystonia is the stronger lateralizing sign.

1.4 1.5 A pragmatic semiologic worksheet

Question	What to document	Interpretive implication
What was the very first symptom?	Exact patient wording, body location, visual field, emotional tone, visceral quality	Best opportunity for onset localization
What was the first visible sign?	Eye/head position, face involvement, limb posture, awareness	Often strongest lateralizing information
How many seconds from onset to each sign?	Latency to version, automatisms, tonic posturing, dysphasia, GTC	Helps distinguish onset from spread
Was awareness preserved?	Can the patient respond, remember, obey commands?	Can help separate frontal, temporal, and hemispheric dominance patterns

Question	What to document	Interpretive implication
What was postictal?	Todd paresis, aphasia, confusion, nose wipe	Often strengthens lateralization
What alternative explanations exist?	Migraine aura, PNES, syncope, movement disorder, sleep parasomnia	Prevents overcalling semiologic localization

CHAPTER 2

Overview of the Uploaded Evidence Base

The reviewed literature includes broad practical reviews, classic semiologic analyses, systematic reviews, meta-analyses, and targeted cohort studies focusing on specific cortical regions and specific signs. The strongest general framework is provided by the broad reviews of Chowdhury et al. and Tufenkjian and Lüders. Subregional depth is added by the SMA/pre-SMA meta-analysis, the posterior cingulate SEEG study, the pediatric hand posture cohort, the head-version timing study, and focused papers on temporal-plus epilepsy, precuneus seizures, ictal grasping, painful parietal seizures, and occipital lobe epilepsy.

Reviewed papers	Main contribution	Relative evidentiary role in this review
Chowdhury et al., 2021	Broad practical lobe-by-lobe semiology guide	Backbone for overall structure and cross-lobe comparison
Tufenkjian & Lüders, 2012	Classifies semiologic signs and explicitly discusses limitations	Backbone for methodology and pitfalls
Buonocore et al., 2026	Systematic review/meta-analysis of SMA and pre-SMA epilepsy	Best summary for mesial frontal motor semiology
Yan et al., 2024	SEEG-based posterior cingulate subregional semiology and stimulation responses	Key source for dPCC, vPCC, and retrosplenial localization
Sivaji et al., 2025	Timing of version and ictal-end head position in secondary generalization	Important for lateralization and timing-based localization
Menderes et al., 2025	Pediatric ictal hand postures	Adds age-specific lateralizing/localizing clues
Khoja et al., 2021	Temporal lobe versus temporal-plus epilepsy	Refines temporal versus temporo-occipital/plus patterns
Other focused papers	Precuneus, occipital, parietal pain, ictal grasping, temporal lobe signs	Supplement specific sign-region correlations

A recurring feature of this evidence base is asymmetry in depth. Frontal, temporal, and cross-cutting lateralizing signs are richly represented. Precuneal, posterior cingulate, and pediatric semiology are more focused but derive from smaller datasets. For some sublobar regions, the review therefore uses strong language only when supported by either systematic synthesis or repeated concordant findings across more than one uploaded paper.

Three additional focused cohort papers are especially helpful for practical nuance in areas the broader reviews mention only briefly. Fotedar et al. (2022) refine the phenomenology of true version in spontaneous seizures; Fayerstein et al. (2020) quantify hyperkinetic seizure patterns across prefrontal, temporal, parietal, and insular onsets; and Hirsch et al. (1998) restore attention to postictal nosewiping as a temporal and ipsilateral side marker. In the expanded discussion below, these papers are used to sharpen the treatment of version, hyperkinetic differential diagnosis, and postictal lateralization.

CHAPTER 3

Frontal Lobe Epilepsy

Frontal lobe epilepsy is consistently described as having seizures characterized by short, often sleep-related, rapidly propagating seizures in which motor behavior dominates the bedside picture. The same connectivity that makes frontal seizures striking also makes them difficult to localize precisely from appearance alone. Elementary motor signs typically arise from precentral or premotor regions, whereas progressively more integrated or semipurposeful behaviors arise from rostral and mesial frontal networks. Thus, frontal semiology must always be read through the lens of both anatomy and speed of spread (Chowdhury et al., 2021; Tufenkjian & Lüders, 2012).

3.1 Primary motor cortex (lateral and medial precentral gyrus)

Overview

Precentral seizures are the clearest examples of pathophysiologic semiology. When the discharge begins within primary motor cortex, the first visible manifestation is usually contralateral clonic activity, sometimes tonic or myoclonic, involving the body part represented in the homunculus (see figure below). Because the motor strip is organized somatotopically, face onset suggests a more lateral precentral region, arm onset an intermediate region, and leg onset a more medial parasagittal location.

Figure 3. EEG seizure onset: face, arm, leg.

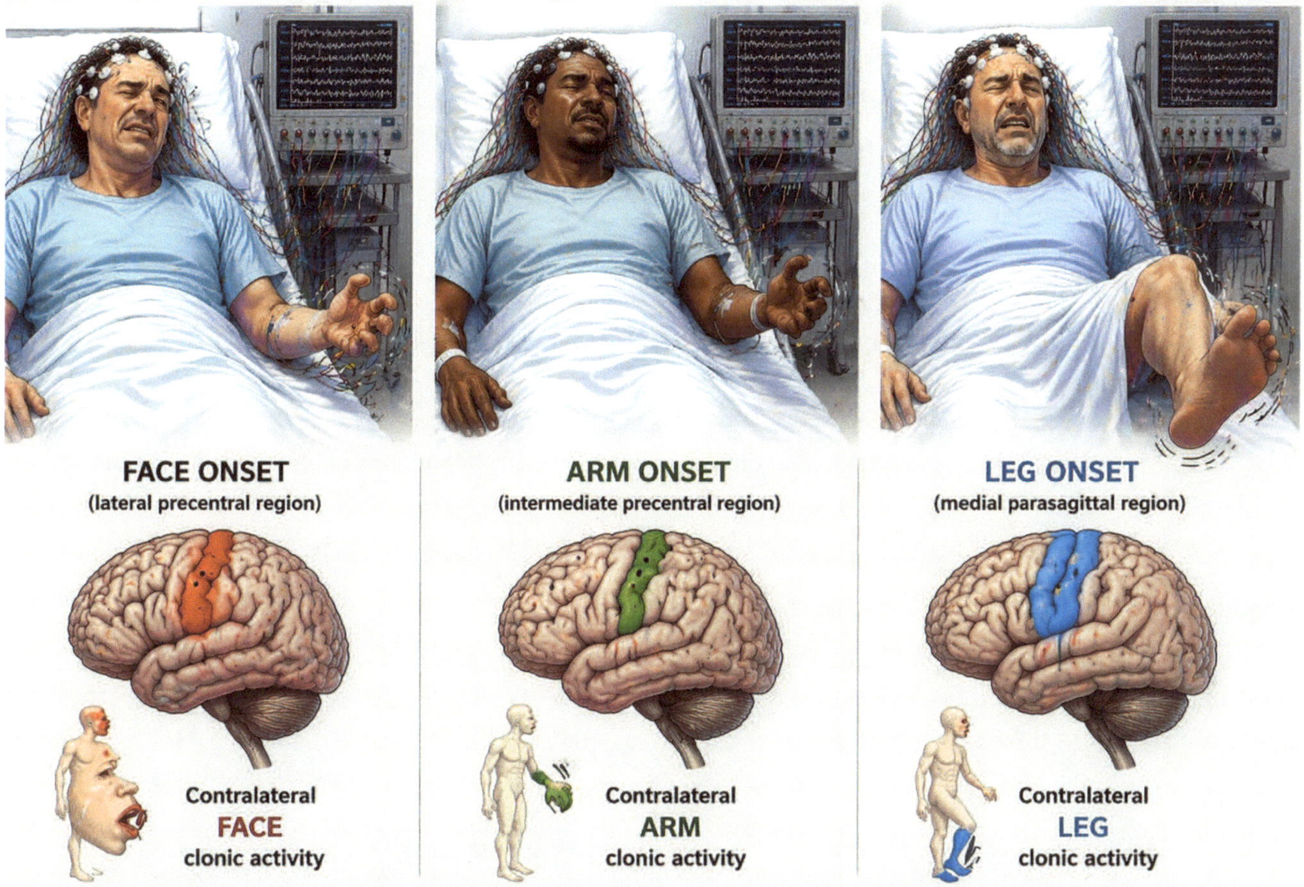

When the discharge begins within primary motor cortex, the first visible manifestation is usually contralateral clonic activity, sometimes tonic or myoclonic, involving the body part represented in the homunculus. Because the motor strip is organized somatotopically, face onset suggests a more lateral precentral region, arm onset an intermediate region, and leg onset a more medial parasagittal location.

Earliest and most localizing features

The most useful pattern is a contralateral focal clonic onset, especially if it is the first unmistakable sign and especially if the clonic activity marches in a Jacksonian fashion. A slow Jacksonian march strongly supports true tangential spread across motor cortex rather than explosive network recruitment.

Usual propagation and semiologic evolution

As the discharge propagates, the seizure may recruit adjacent precentral or supplementary motor regions, producing tonic posturing, fencing, or secondary generalization. This later evolution should not erase the localizing value of the initial clonic onset.

Lateralizing implications

Unilateral clonic motor onset is strongly lateralizing to the contralateral hemisphere. If the earliest sign is clearly unilateral face clonus or arm clonus, the side of onset is usually secure even when scalp EEG is partially obscured by movement.

Main pitfalls and differential considerations

Later tonic posturing or version can tempt the observer to overcall SMA or frontal eye field onset. The practical correction is to privilege the initial contralateral clonus over the later motor sequence. Movement artifact can also limit scalp EEG correlation in these seizures.

3.2 Supplementary motor area (SMA) and pre-supplementary motor area

Overview

The mesial superior frontal region is one of the best studied frontal subregions in the uploaded set because it is covered both in the practical review and in a dedicated 2026 systematic review/meta-analysis. Across different reviewed papers, SMA epilepsy is characterized by brief, abrupt, often sleep-related seizures with bilateral but asymmetric tonic posturing. The classic pattern is contralateral arm extension with ipsilateral arm flexion, often referred to as fencing posture, sometimes accompanied by contralateral head and eye deviation and sometimes preceded by sensory phenomena such as tingling or a sense of tightness.

Earliest and most localizing features

The earliest and most useful sign is unilateral or asymmetric tonic posturing that begins at onset, particularly when coupled with the classic upper-limb asymmetry. (see fence posturing in the following 2 figures) and figure of four the third figure.

Figure. Sudden onset of fencing posture in a patient with right supplementary motor area epilepsy.

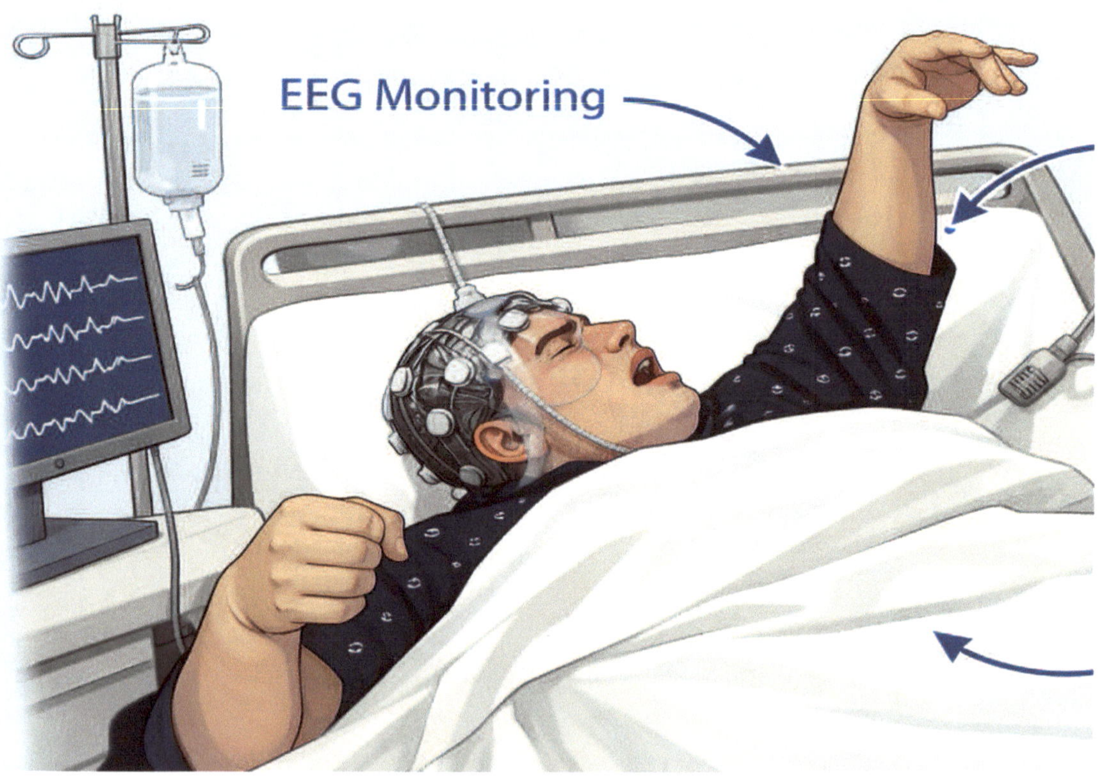

Figure 4. Figure. Sudden onset of fencing posture with right arm extension in a patient with left supplementary motor area epilepsy.

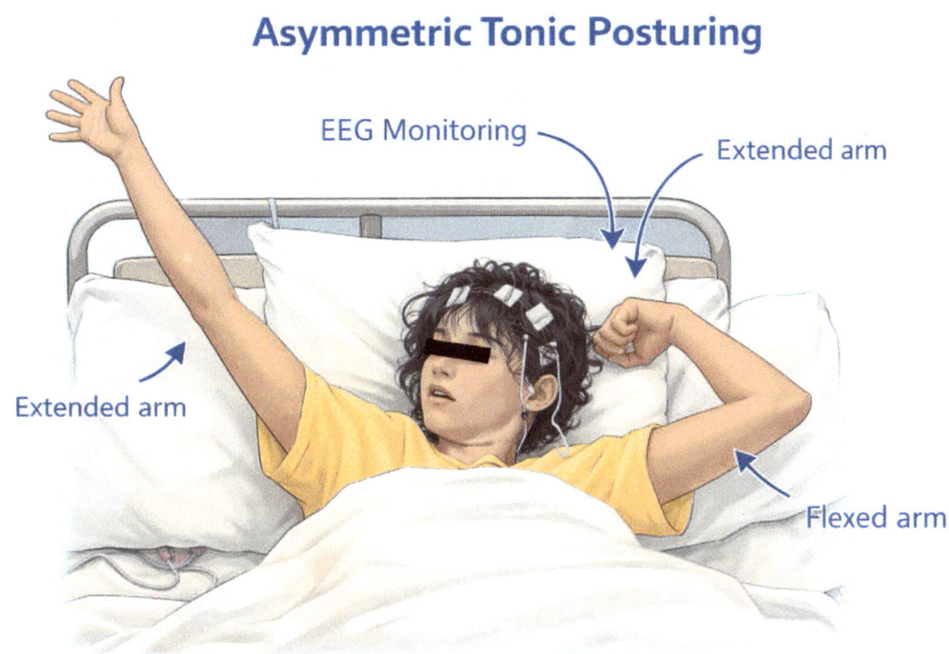

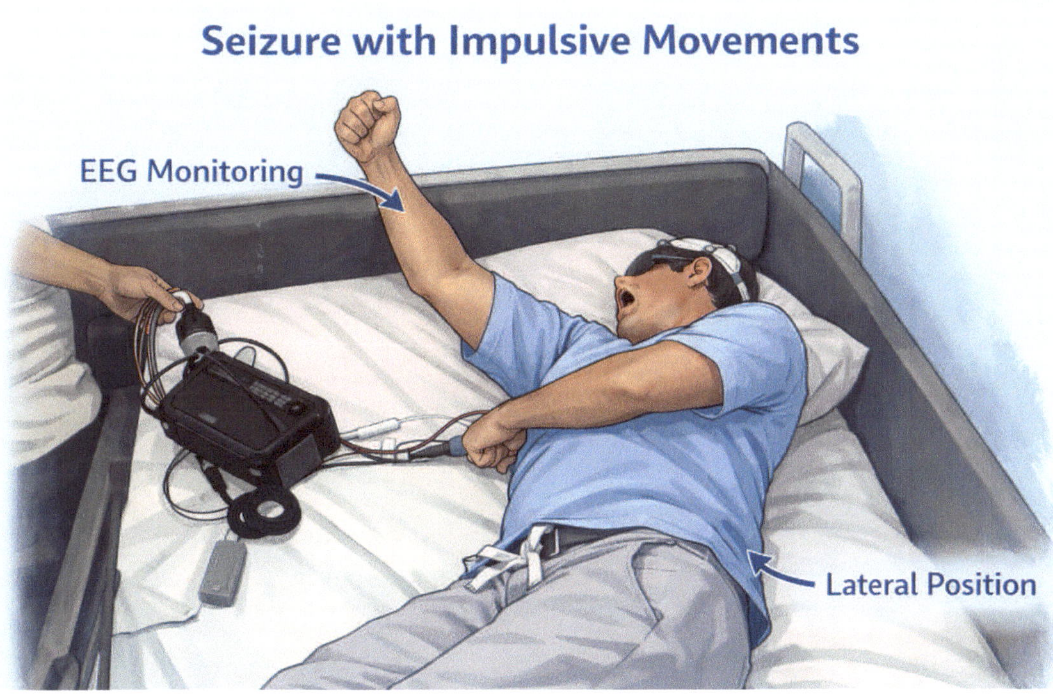

Figure 6. Figure-of-four sign in a patient with left supplementary motor area epilepsy.

In the 2026 meta-analysis, asymmetric tonic posturing was the most frequent ictal feature, present in 47% of patients, followed by automatisms in 25%, version in 23%, loss of consciousness in 19%, sensory phenomena in 11%, and speech arrest/inhibition in 10%. These numbers are important because they show that even the 'classic' SMA sign is present in fewer than half of confirmed cases; absence of fencing or asymmetric tonic posture does not exclude SMA epilepsy.

Usual propagation and semiologic evolution

SMA seizures may remain relatively restricted, but they often generalize rapidly or recruit adjacent premotor, motor, or cingulate networks. This explains why some patients develop version, bilateral tonic-clonic progression, or less specific frontal motor patterns. The pre-SMA remains more weakly characterized in the uploaded evidence; the 2026 meta-analysis specifically notes that the literature does not yet allow a confident separation of pre-SMA from SMA-proper on semiology alone.

Lateralizing implications

Asymmetric tonic posturing and fencing posture are typically contralateral to the side of onset when interpreted by the extended arm. Version that begins early in the sequence also usually points contralaterally. However, because the symptomatogenic zone of tonic posturing can be recruited by spread from parietal or occipital regions, lateralization should be combined with the total sequence rather than used in isolation.

Main pitfalls and differential considerations

The key pitfall is false SMA localization from extrafrontal seizures that propagate to mesial frontal motor areas. The practical guide explicitly warns that parietal and occipital seizures can produce asymmetric tonic posturing after spread to the SMA. Thus, an aura or a very early sensory/visual symptom preceding the tonic phase should lower confidence in pure SMA onset (see figure below). Another pitfall is the frequent nonlocalizing scalp EEG of mesial frontal seizures.

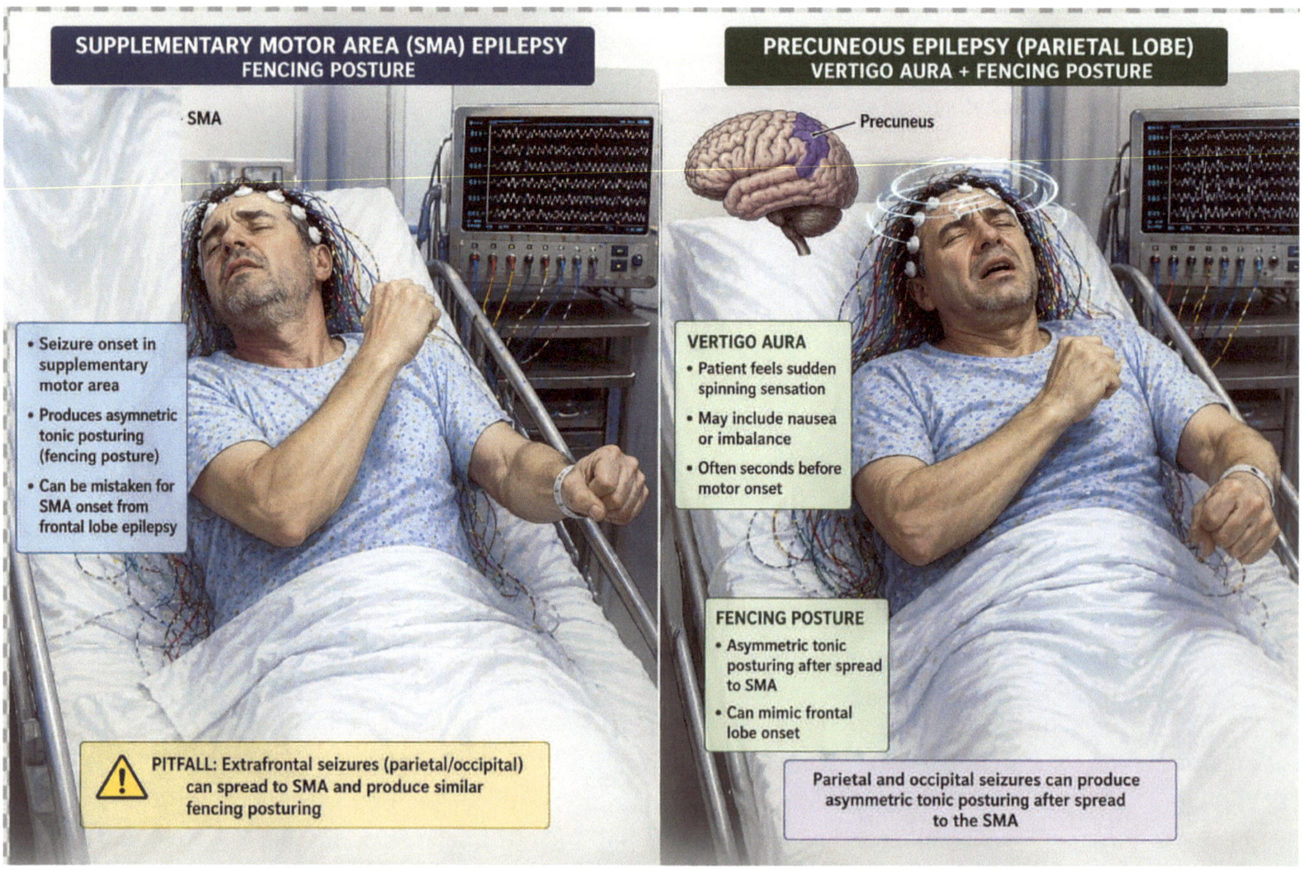

Figure 7. Figure. Asymmetric tonic posturing in two patients. The first patient has supplementary motor area epilepsy. The second has parietal lobe epilepsy with precuneus onset demonstrated by SEEG.

3.3 Frontal eye field and dorsolateral frontal cortex

Overview

The dorsolateral frontal region, particularly when the frontal eye field is involved, is classically associated with early versive head and eye deviation. Version is a symptomatogenic sign of frontal eye field recruitment rather than a direct marker of frontal onset per se.

Earliest and most localizing features

The most localizing situation is very early version, especially when the head and eyes are forcibly and unnaturally driven to one side with neck extension. The distinction between true version and merely natural head turning is essential; the bedside observer must insist on forcefulness, sustained deviation, and unnatural appearance.

Usual propagation and semiologic evolution

If version occurs early, especially close to onset, frontal onset becomes more likely than temporal or occipital onset. The timing paper by Sivaji et al. adds an important nuance: latency from seizure onset to version has localizing significance. Version appeared earliest in frontal lobe epilepsy (mean 24.1 seconds), later in temporal epilepsy (46.7 seconds), and latest in occipital epilepsy (77.8 seconds). Version within 15 seconds had a positive predictive value of 85.7% for frontal onset.

Figure 8. Seizure version timing and localization.

EARLY VERSION SUGGESTS FRONTAL ONSET

If version occurs early, especially close to onset, frontal onset becomes more likely than temporal or occipital onset. The timing paper by Sivaji et al. adds an important nuance: latency from seizure onset to version has localizing significance.

TIMING MATTERS

Version within 15 seconds had a positive predictive value of 85.7% for frontal onset.

FRONTAL LOBE EPILEPSY
Earliest Version
Mean latency: 24.1 seconds

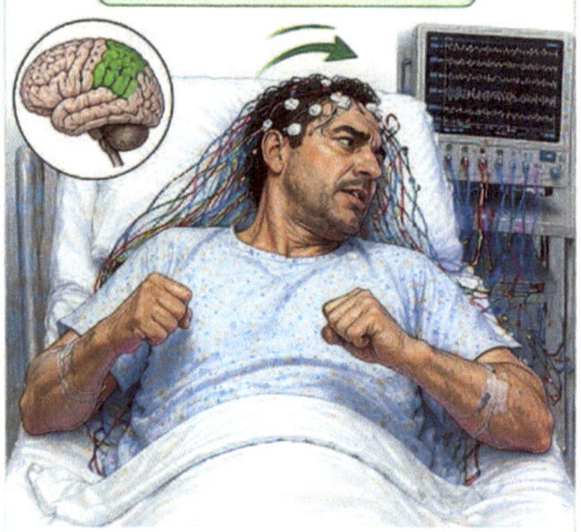

Version to the contralateral side occurs early, mean 24.1 seconds after seizure onset.

TEMPORAL LOBE EPILEPSY
Later Version
Mean latency: 46.7 seconds

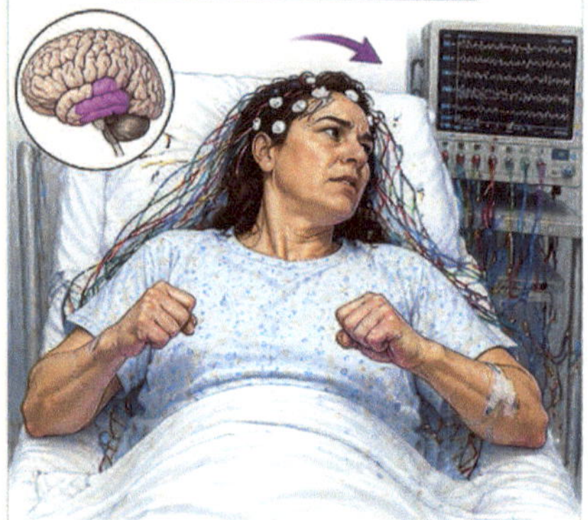

Version to the contralateral side occurs later, mean 46.7 seconds after seizure onset.

OCCIPITAL LOBE EPILEPSY
Latest Version
Mean latency: 77.8 seconds

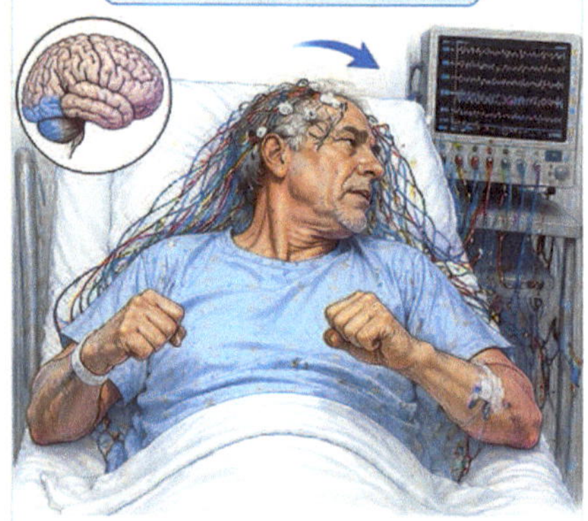

Version to the contralateral side occurs latest, mean 77.8 seconds after seizure onset.

FENCING POSTURE

All patients show asymmetric tonic posturing with arm flexion and adduction, a common sign in focal seizures.

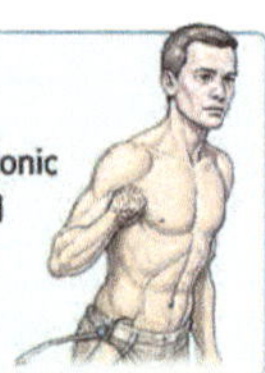

EPILEPSY TYPE	MEAN LATENCY TO VERSION	LOCALIZING SIGNIFICANCE
Frontal Lobe	24.1 seconds	Earliest → Most likely frontal onset
Temporal Lobe	46.7 seconds	Intermediate
Occipital Lobe	77.8 seconds	Latest → Less likely frontal onset

VERSION WITHIN 15 SECONDS = 85.7% POSITIVE PREDICTIVE VALUE FOR FRONTAL ONSET

Lateralizing implications

The direction of early true version is strongly lateralizing to the contralateral hemisphere. The complementary 2025 study also identified a late ictal-end head position, opposite to the initial version, that was always ipsilateral to the epileptogenic zone in the subset with complete three-stage head evolution.

Main pitfalls and differential considerations

Version has high lateralizing value but limited lobe localization if timing is ignored. Frontal and extrafrontal seizures can both recruit the frontal eye field. Nonversive head turning, scanning, or natural repositioning should not be overinterpreted. In practice, the value of version rises when it is very early, unmistakably forced, and paired with other concordant lateralizing signs such as figure-of-four or unilateral dystonia.

3.4 Orbitofrontal and frontopolar cortex

Overview

The orbitofrontal and frontopolar regions often generate impaired-awareness seizures with automatisms or complex motor behavior rather than simple elementary signs. Orbitofrontal seizures may include autonomic symptoms such as tachycardia and occasional olfactory aura. Frontopolar seizures may begin with impaired awareness before developing more obvious motor features.

Earliest and most localizing features

Unlike precentral or calcarine cortex, orbitofrontal and frontopolar regions rarely declare themselves with a single pathognomonic onset sign. The most informative clue is usually the overall pattern: abrupt impaired awareness, complex or semipurposeful behaviors, relative paucity of a specific sensory aura, and sometimes rapid progression into a more obvious frontal motor syndrome.

Usual propagation and semiologic evolution

These seizures often spread quickly to mesial frontal or SMA networks, at which point tonic posturing or hypermotor behavior becomes visible. Because scalp EEG can be nonlocalizing for deep orbitofrontal onset, the visible seizure may appear to begin only after the discharge has already spread.

Lateralizing implications

Lateralization from orbitofrontal semiology alone is usually modest unless accompanied by early unilateral motor signs or true version. Olfactory aura may suggest orbitofrontal involvement but is not exclusive to it because mesial temporal and insular structures can produce similar symptoms.

Main pitfalls and differential considerations

The main pitfall is false non-epileptic classification. Rapid, bizarre, sleep-related, or poorly localizable orbitofrontal seizures can be mistaken for parasomnia or psychogenic events when scalp EEG is unrevealing. Another pitfall is assuming that hypermotor evolution automatically implies mesial frontal rather than orbitofrontal origin.

Evidence anchor

Chowdhury et al., 2021 provide the clearest practical summary, while the more general frontal lobe framework in Tufenkjian & Lüders helps explain why orbitofrontal semiology is often less anatomically pure.

3.5 Mesial prefrontal and anterior cingulate regions within the frontal network

Overview

Seizures involving ventromedial prefrontal and anterior cingulate regions occupy the borderland between frontal lobe epilepsy and cingulate network epilepsy. The practical features highlighted in the uploaded papers include fear, screaming, vocalization, autonomic activation, hypermotor behavior, and, in some patients, forced thinking.

Figure 9. Illustrative semiology figure.

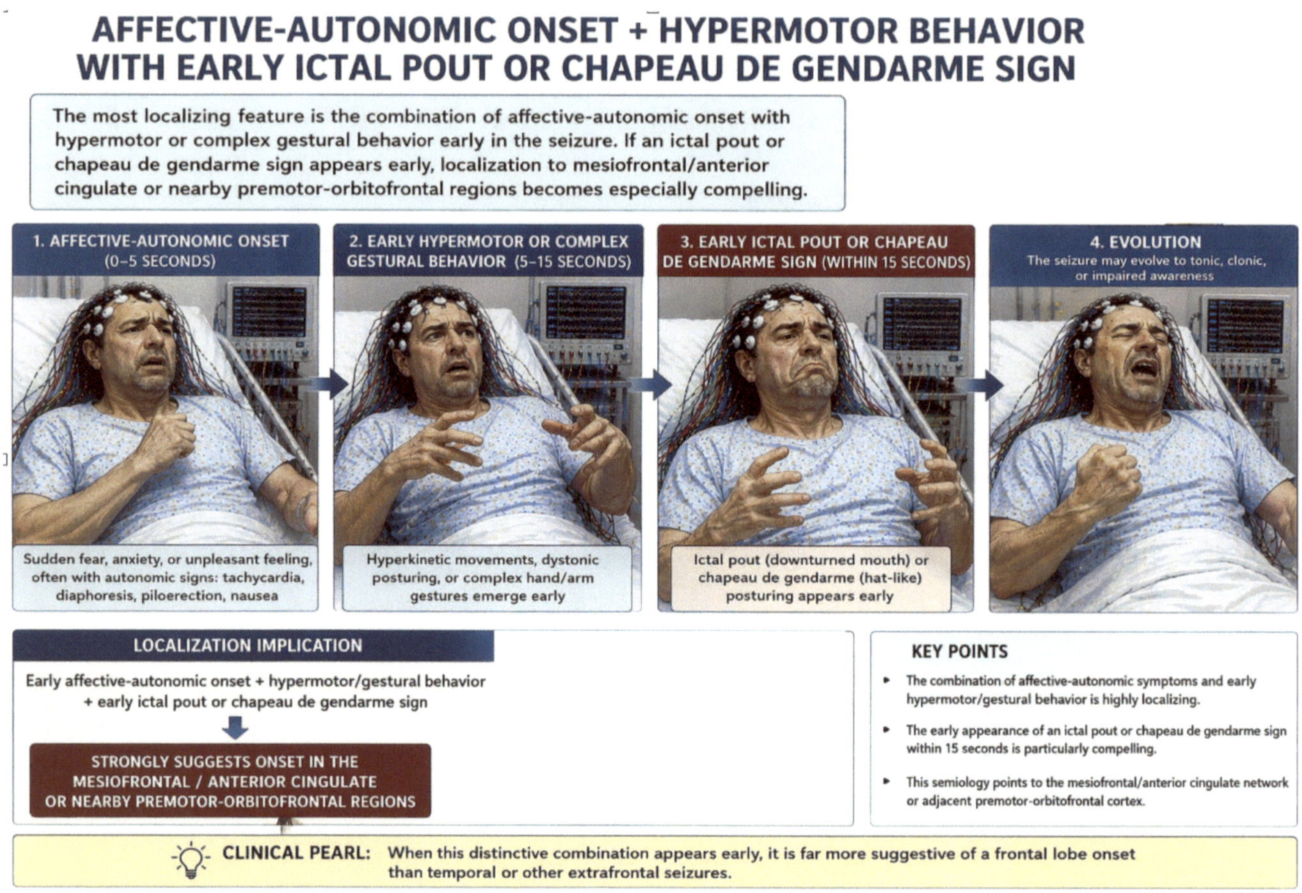

Earliest and most localizing features

The most localizing feature is the combination of affective-autonomic onset with hypermotor or complex gestural behavior early in the seizure. If an ictal pout or chapeau de gendarme sign appears early, localization to mesiofrontal/anterior cingulate or nearby premotor-orbitofrontal regions becomes especially compelling.

Usual propagation and semiologic evolution

These seizures frequently generalize or recruit wider frontal motor networks, producing a more dramatic motor phase than the onset itself might suggest. Some reported anterior cingulate cases have simpler motor features and more frequent generalization, particularly in infiltrative lesional epilepsy.

Lateralizing implications

Lateralization is usually derived from accompanying motor signs rather than from the affective or vocal component itself. An early contralateral tonic or clonic asymmetry, or concordant version, is more trustworthy than fear or vocalization for the side of onset.

Main pitfalls and differential considerations

The pitfall is overcalling temporal lobe onset because fear is present. Although fear can be a mesial temporal experiential aura, in anterior cingulate seizures it is usually embedded in a more explosively motor and autonomic syndrome. The observer should therefore separate isolated experiential fear from fear plus hypermotor behavior plus screaming or vocalization.

3.6 Frontal operculum, Broca region, and negative motor areas

Overview

Frontal opercular seizures are notable for face-predominant clonic motor phenomena, articulation difficulty, laryngeal symptoms, and hypersalivation. Dominant inferior frontal involvement may produce dysphasia, while negative motor area recruitment may produce focal atonic or akinetic phenomena.

Earliest and most localizing features

The earliest localizing cluster is unilateral face clonus with speech disturbance, hypersalivation, or anarthria-like difficulty, particularly when these features emerge before a more widespread motor phase.

Usual propagation and semiologic evolution

Because the frontal operculum lies close to insular and perisylvian networks, spread is common and the seizure may quickly acquire visceral, somatosensory, or automotor features. Negative motor areas may instead produce arrest of movement or apparent apraxic inability to move despite preserved awareness.

Lateralizing implications

Dysphasia lateralizes to the dominant hemisphere but has only limited localizing precision within the frontal-temporal language network. Speech arrest must be distinguished from true aphasic impairment. Akinetic or atonic phenomena by themselves are not strong lobe localizers unless the sequence and preserved awareness strongly support a frontal negative motor mechanism.

Main pitfalls and differential considerations

The main pitfall is confusion with insular onset because frontal opercular and insular seizures share laryngeal, salivatory, and speech-related semiology. Another pitfall is mistaking negative motor or akinetic seizures for psychogenic freezing or non-epileptic inability to move.

Evidence anchor

The practical guide by Chowdhury et al. is the most specific uploaded source for this region; Tufenkjian & Lüders provide the conceptual distinction between akinetic, atonic, and other negative motor phenomena.

3.7 Frontal lobe synthesis

Taken together, the uploaded papers support a useful frontal rule: the more elementary the onset sign, the more likely the cortical onset is close to primary or supplementary motor systems; the more integrated, semipurposeful, emotional, or bizarre the behavior, the more likely the observer is seeing rapid recruitment of broader frontal networks. Frontal seizures are usually brief, often arise in sleep, propagate quickly, and may be clinically dramatic despite poor scalp EEG localization. They are best interpreted by identifying the first motor vector in the sequence and resisting the temptation to over-weight later generalization.

Clinical takeaway

- Best onset clue: identify the first motor vector rather than the final motor storm.
- Best lateralizers: early focal clonus, tonic asymmetry, and true early version.
- Common trap: propagated posterior or temporal seizures masquerading as primary frontal onset.

- Escalate to invasive EEG early when orbitofrontal, mesial frontal, or deep-network onset remains plausible.

CHAPTER 4

Temporal Lobe Epilepsy

Temporal lobe epilepsy is the commonest focal epilepsy in surgical cohorts and the most richly developed semiologic tradition in the uploaded set. The central bedside pattern is familiar—behavioral arrest, oral and manual automatisms, impaired awareness, and postictal confusion—but the practical value lies in separating mesial temporal, lateral neocortical temporal, temporal pole, and temporal-plus patterns. The onset aura, the nature of early autonomic or auditory symptoms, language involvement, and the timing of later motor signs are particularly helpful.

4.1 Mesial temporal lobe (hippocampus-dominant pattern)

Overview

Mesial temporal seizures classically begin with experiential or visceral aura and evolve into behavioral arrest, oral and manual automatisms, impaired awareness, and postictal confusion. In the uploaded practical guide, abdominal rising or epigastric discomfort is the signature onset phenomenon, while déjà vu, jamais vu, and fear are additional high-yield experiential auras.

Earliest and most localizing features

The strongest localizing pattern is an abdominal aura, especially one that evolves into an automotor seizure. In the dataset cited by Chowdhury et al., an abdominal aura carried a probability of 74% for temporal lobe epilepsy, and when it evolved into an automotor seizure the probability rose to 98%. In a large intracranial temporal series, abdominal aura and experiential phenomena such as fear, déjà vu, and jamais vu preferentially indicated mesial temporal onset.

Usual propagation and semiologic evolution

The usual evolution is from aura to behavioral arrest, then oral/manual automatisms, then impaired awareness. Seizures are often longer than frontal seizures, commonly lasting 30 seconds to 2 minutes or longer, with a more gradual onset and more prolonged postictal confusion. Before secondary generalization, mesial temporal seizures may acquire version or a figure-of-four posture, but these late motor signs should be interpreted as lateralizing spread rather than proof of frontal onset.

Lateralizing implications

Several classic lateralizing signs remain useful. Unilateral dystonic posturing is contralateral to seizure onset. Early head version is also contralateral. In bilateral tonic-clonic evolution, the last clonic jerk is often ipsilateral to onset. Preserved awareness during an automotor seizure favors the non-dominant hemisphere. Ictal speech also tends to suggest non-dominant temporal involvement, whereas ictal or postictal dysphasia supports dominant hemisphere involvement.

Main pitfalls and differential considerations

The major pitfall is reciprocal spread between mesial and neocortical temporal cortex. Once the seizure reaches lateral temporal, insular, or frontal networks, the bedside pattern can change dramatically. Another pitfall is to overinterpret nonspecific emotional symptoms as mesial temporal when they may instead reflect anterior cingulate or posterior cingulate spread.

4.2 Amygdala-predominant mesial temporal pattern

Overview

Within mesial temporal epilepsy, amygdalar involvement tends to amplify autonomic and affective semiology. The uploaded practical guide highlights early flushing, tachycardia, and apnoea as especially important when present at onset or very early in the course.

Earliest and most localizing features

The most localizing clue is early autonomic activation—particularly apnoea and tachycardia—embedded within a mesial temporal sequence. In a patient whose seizure begins with fear or visceral aura and then quickly shows apnoea or marked tachycardia before typical temporal automatisms, amygdalar participation becomes especially plausible.

Usual propagation and semiologic evolution

As the seizure evolves, the pattern usually merges with the broader mesial temporal syndrome of behavioral arrest and automatisms. Because hippocampus and amygdala are densely connected, the bedside observer is rarely able to separate them with certainty from semiology alone unless the autonomic pattern is especially conspicuous.

Lateralizing implications

Figure 10. Autonomic signs by themselves have modest lateralizing power. The side of onset is better inferred from accompanying unilateral dystonia, version, figure-of-four, and postictal asymmetry.

Main pitfalls and differential considerations

The pitfall is assuming that all strong autonomic onset must be insular. The anterior insula and amygdala overlap considerably in visceral and autonomic semiology. The best discriminator is the total sequence: insular onset more often combines visceral sensations with broad somatosensory or laryngeal phenomena, whereas amygdalar/mesial temporal onset more often merges into classic automotor temporal seizures (see figure 10 below).

Figure 10. Insular onset vs mesial temporal lobe onset.

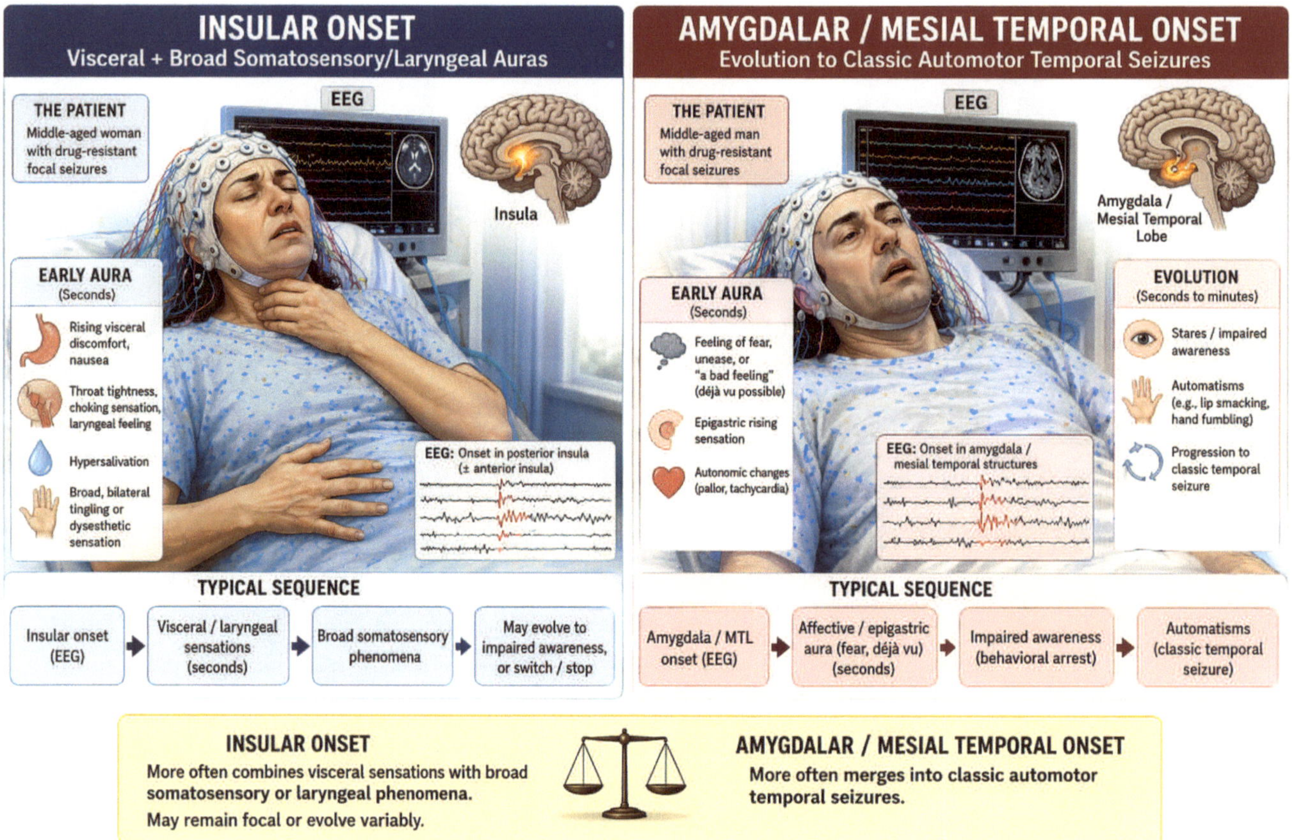

4.3 Lateral temporal neocortex and Heschl gyrus

Overview

Lateral neocortical temporal seizures have greater semiologic overlap with temporoparietal and temporo-occipital cortex than mesial temporal seizures do. The most useful onset clues are simple auditory aura, vertiginous symptoms, early language disturbance, or less commonly complex auditory distortions or visual illusions.

Earliest and most localizing features

The earliest and most localizing sign is an elementary auditory aura—buzzing, ringing, or humming—suggesting primary auditory cortex or Heschl gyrus. When unilateral, such an auditory aura lateralizes contralaterally. Ictal dysphasia early in the seizure suggests dominant hemisphere lateral temporal involvement. Vertiginous symptoms suggest extension into temporoparietal vestibular cortex.

Usual propagation and semiologic evolution

Lateral temporal seizures are typically shorter than mesial temporal seizures and more likely to propagate early into frontal regions, producing complex motor features or more rapid evolution to bilateral tonic-clonic seizures. Because reciprocal mesial-lateral temporal connections are strong, many seizures rapidly lose their anatomically pure onset appearance.

Lateralizing implications

The side of onset is supported by unilateral auditory aura, early aphasic disturbance in the dominant hemisphere, contralateral dystonia if present, and version if it appears early enough to retain lateralizing value. Peri-ictal drinking, spitting, vomiting, or urge to urinate point toward a non-dominant temporal focus but do not by themselves define lateral neocortical versus mesial onset.

Main pitfalls and differential considerations

The main pitfall is false mesial temporal labeling when early auditory or vestibular symptoms are overlooked and the observer anchors on later automatisms. Another pitfall is confusion with temporal-plus or temporo-occipital onset because the same seizure may include both auditory and visual/vertiginous features.

4.4 Temporoparietal and temporo-occipital border zones

Overview

The temporoparietal-occipital border is less a single lobe than a convergence zone in which auditory, visual, vestibular, and language networks intersect. The literature repeatedly identify vertigo, visual hallucinations or illusions, and language disturbance as clues that the seizure is not a straightforward mesial temporal event.

Earliest and most localizing features

The earliest localizing signs here are vestibular symptoms, visual illusions, complex visual hallucinations, and mixed auditory-visual auras. When dominant hemisphere language cortex is nearby, reading and expressive deficits may also appear early.

Usual propagation and semiologic evolution

These seizures often evolve into temporal automatisms or impaired awareness because spread to mesial temporal structures is common. That evolution can make the final seizure look mesial temporal unless the onset semiology is preserved carefully.

Lateralizing implications

Lateralization follows the sign itself more than the border-zone label. Hemifield visual phenomena lateralize contralaterally; unilateral auditory aura is contralateral; early aphasia points to the dominant hemisphere.

Main pitfalls and differential considerations

The key pitfall is calling every automotor seizure 'temporal' without recognizing that the onset may actually be at the temporo-occipital or temporoparietal junction. A practical way to avoid this error is to ask whether the aura is purely experiential-visceral or whether it has a sensory-perceptual quality that better fits a posterior network.

4.5 Temporal pole

Overview

Temporal pole seizures are not semeiologically identical to either hippocampal or lateral superior temporal seizures. In the literature reviewed they are associated with earlier loss of consciousness and more frequent hypermotor features than classic mesial temporal seizures.

Earliest and most localizing features

The most useful clue is the mismatch between a seizure that still appears 'temporal' in aura content or automotor evolution yet loses awareness unusually early or acquires early hypermotor features.

Usual propagation and semiologic evolution

Propagation from the temporal pole can quickly recruit mesial temporal, lateral temporal, and frontal networks. This explains why temporal pole seizures may blur the boundary between temporal and frontal semiology.

Lateralizing implications

Lateralization generally relies on the same classic temporal signs as elsewhere: unilateral dystonia, early version, language dominance phenomena, and postictal asymmetries.

Main pitfalls and differential considerations

The pitfall is false frontal localization due to hypermotor features. If a seizure begins with temporal aura but becomes hypermotor early, temporal pole origin should stay in the differential.

4.6 Temporal-plus epilepsy

Overview

Temporal-plus epilepsy refers to seizures that involve the temporal lobe together with adjacent extratemporal structures such as the temporo-occipital, insular, orbitofrontal, or parietal/perisylvian network. Avoid overly simple temporal labeling.

Earliest and most localizing features

Visual hallucinations and vertigo are especially associated with temporal-plus epilepsy, fitting the idea that posterior temporal or temporo-occipital participation modifies the onset experience. By contrast, early-onset manual automatisms, oral automatisms, late-onset dystonic posture, and late head version were more significant for conventional temporal lobe epilepsy without meaningful additional lateralizing value.

Usual propagation and semiologic evolution

The semiologic evolution of temporal-plus seizures is therefore often 'hybrid': an event may begin with visual, vestibular, auditory, or affective symptoms and then pass through a temporal automotor phase. This pattern should not be forced into a purely mesial temporal model simply because automatisms are present later.

Lateralizing implications

Lateralization in temporal-plus epilepsy remains sign-based rather than syndrome-based. A hemifield visual aura is still contralateral, unilateral auditory aura is still contralateral, and dominant language disturbance still points toward the dominant hemisphere.

Main pitfalls and differential considerations

The main pitfall is under-recognition. A seizure that starts with vertigo or visual hallucination and then becomes automotor may be misclassified as mesial temporal if the observer relies only on the middle phase.

In presurgical patients, this mistake matters because temporal-plus localization may explain temporal surgery failures or unexpected invasive EEG findings.

4.7 Temporal lobe synthesis

The most useful temporal heuristic from the uploaded literature is simple: the aura usually tells you more than the later motor sequence. Visceral-experiential onset supports mesial temporal epilepsy. Simple auditory onset supports lateral temporal/Heschl gyrus. Vertiginous, mixed visual-auditory, or hybrid posterior sensory onset raises temporal-plus or temporo-occipital involvement. Later automatisms, dystonia, and version remain valuable but should be interpreted as part of the evolving sequence rather than as isolated region markers.

Clinical takeaway

- Best onset clue: the aura usually localizes better than the later motor phase.
- Best lateralizers: unilateral dystonia, early version, and dominance-related language signs.
- Common trap: temporal-plus or posterior onset mislabeled as straightforward mesial temporal epilepsy.
- Escalate to invasive EEG when visual, vestibular, auditory, or early hypermotor features complicate the temporal narrative.

CHAPTER 5

Insular and Operculo-Insular Epilepsy

The insula is one of the most deceptive cortical regions in semiology because it is deeply situated, heavily connected, and capable of producing visceral, somatosensory, autonomic, language, and motor phenomena. Insular onset is best approached not by looking for a single pathognomonic sign, but by identifying the unusual combination of visceral-autonomic and somatosensory features, especially when they involve broad territories or the perioral region and then evolve rapidly into temporal or frontal behavior.

5.1 Anterior insula

Overview

Anterior insular seizures are especially associated with viscerosensory and autonomic onset. The practical approach is to consider abdominal aura, laryngeal constriction, nausea, hypersalivation, sweating, and related visceral discomfort as the most characteristic early clues.

Earliest and most localizing features

Figure 11. Illustrative semiology figure.

The most localizing pattern is a complex visceral-autonomic onset that cannot be fully explained by a simple mesial temporal epigastric aura: for example, rising visceral discomfort plus throat tightness, choking-like laryngeal sensation, hypersalivation, nausea, and broad somatic discomfort (see illustration below).

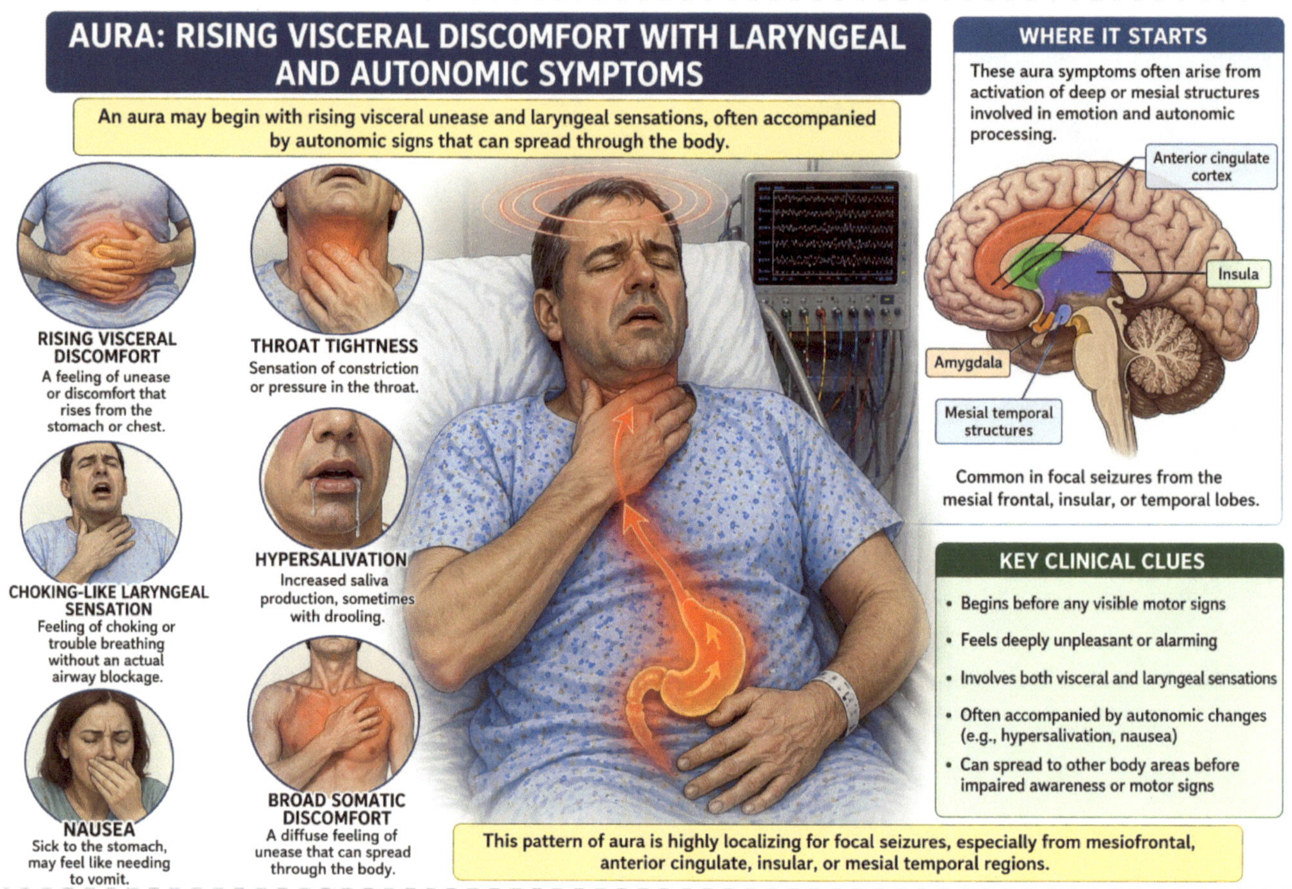

Usual propagation and semiologic evolution

Because the insula rapidly propagates to mesial temporal and frontal systems, the seizure often evolves into automotor behavior, hypermotor activity, tonic posturing, or altered awareness. This rapid evolution explains why purely bedside diagnosis of insular epilepsy is difficult.

Lateralizing implications

Lateralization is less robust than localization by syndrome. If unilateral somatosensory or motor signs emerge early, they should be interpreted according to their usual contralateral rules. Autonomic symptoms themselves rarely lateralize reliably.

Main pitfalls and differential considerations

The main pitfall is false mesial temporal localization because abdominal aura is also common in hippocampal seizures. The distinction lies in the richness of the bodily and laryngeal component, the larger body territory affected, and the frequent admixture of somatosensory features.

5.2 Posterior insula

Overview

Posterior insular seizures are more strongly associated with painful, burning, electric, tingling, or broad somatosensory sensations. The practical guide and the classic review both note that painful sensations more likely arise from posterior insula than from anterior insula.

Earliest and most localizing features

The most localizing onset pattern is a painful or dysesthetic aura that is broad, perioral, bilateral, or otherwise larger in territory than typical primary sensory cortex seizures. Posterior insular onset may also produce tingling or shock-like sensations that are not neatly restricted to a small somatotopic segment.

Figure 12. Illustrative semiology figure.

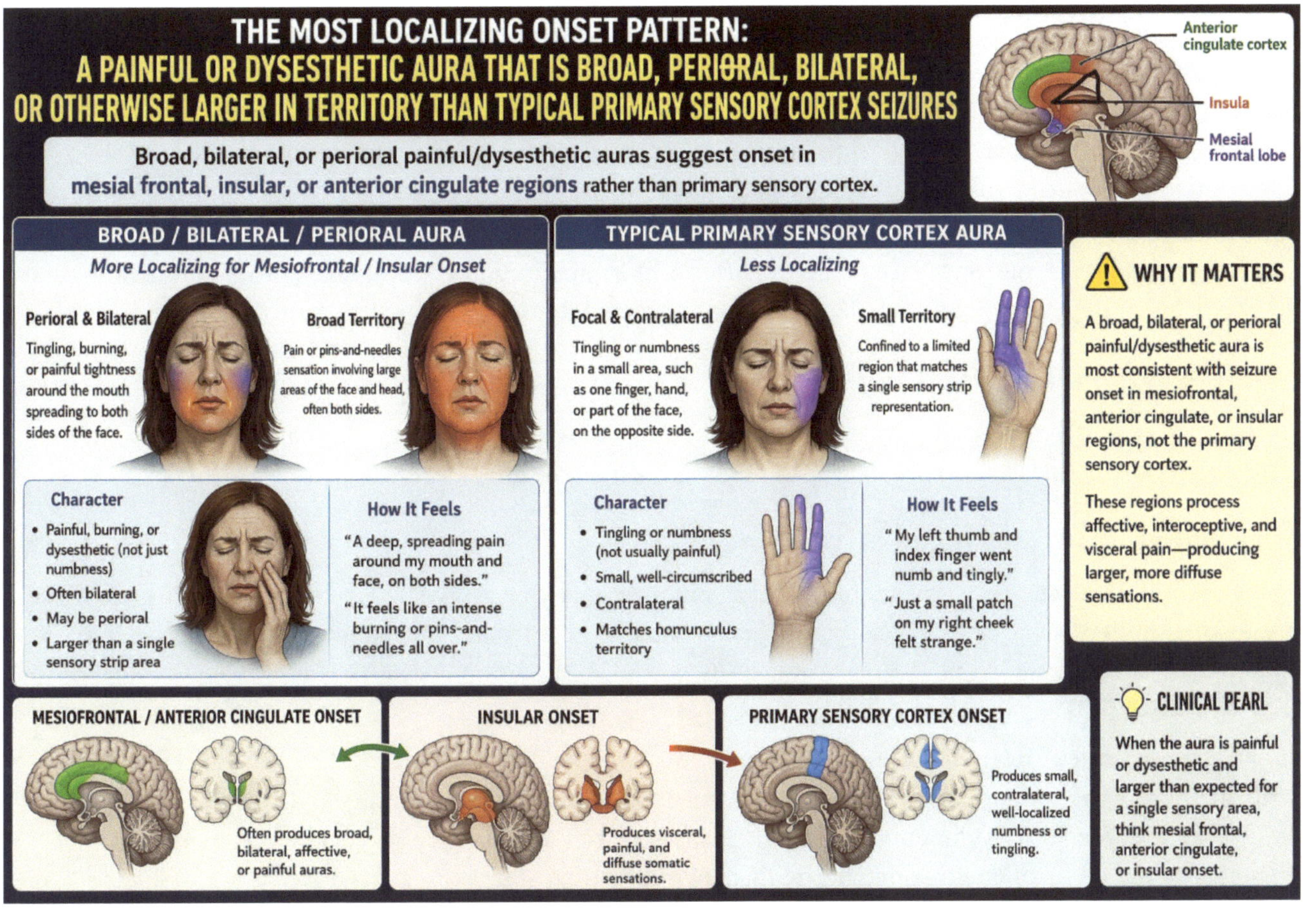

Usual propagation and semiologic evolution

As spread occurs, the seizure may evolve into complex motor activity, altered awareness, or temporal/frontal-like behavior. The broader the sensory territory and the more rapidly the seizure acquires visceral or motor complexity, the more plausible insular participation becomes.

Lateralizing implications

If the sensory aura is clearly unilateral and focal, lateralization still follows the usual contralateral rule. However, bilateral or ipsilateral sensory spread is not uncommon in insular seizures and therefore reduces confidence in standard somatotopic lateralization.

Main pitfalls and differential considerations

The pitfall is confusion with primary sensory or secondary sensory cortex seizures. The best clue favoring insula is that insular sensory symptoms tend to affect larger, less tidy body territories, more often involve perioral regions, and more often evolve into complex motor phenomena.

5.3 Operculo-insular and perisylvian overlap

Overview

Many clinically relevant seizures do not respect a clean border between insula and adjacent opercular cortex. Frontal opercular, parietal opercular, and insular seizures can all produce mixed laryngeal, salivatory, face-predominant, speech-related, and sensory symptoms.

Earliest and most localizing features

The most localizing semiologic clue here is the coexistence of laryngeal or oral symptoms with salivatory features, speech disturbance, and a broad or unusual somatosensory aura. Such combinations should prompt explicit consideration of an operculo-insular network rather than forced assignment to a single lobe.

Usual propagation and semiologic evolution

These seizures may evolve into face clonus, anarthria-like impairment, visceral discomfort, and later automatisms or hypermotor activity, depending on which neighboring cortex is recruited first.

Lateralizing implications

Lateralization is driven primarily by the associated unilateral motor or sensory sign rather than by hypersalivation or speech arrest alone.

Main pitfalls and differential considerations

The main pitfall is categorical overconfidence. In practice, many perisylvian seizures require invasive EEG because semiology alone cannot cleanly separate anterior insula, frontal operculum, and parietal operculum.

5.4 Insular/perisylvian synthesis

If one practical rule is retained for insular epilepsy, it should be this: think of insula when a seizure begins with an unusual mixture of body-internal sensation, autonomic activation, laryngeal discomfort, salivation, and broad somatosensory symptoms, especially if the seizure then quickly masquerades as temporal or frontal. The pattern is often more diagnostic than any individual sign.

Clinical takeaway

- Best onset clue: a mixed visceral-autonomic-laryngeal or broad dysesthetic onset pattern.
- Best lateralizers: accompanying unilateral motor or sensory asymmetry rather than the aura alone.
- Common trap: false mesial temporal or frontal labeling after rapid spread.
- Escalate to invasive EEG when operculo-insular overlap is a serious possibility.

CHAPTER 6

Parietal Lobe Epilepsy

Parietal lobe epilepsy is one of the most semeiologically diverse and diagnostically difficult focal epilepsies. The practical reviews repeatedly emphasize that the symptomatogenic zone may be distant from the true onset zone because the parietal lobe is richly connected with frontal, temporal, occipital, insular, and cingulate networks. This is why parietal epilepsy is both underdiagnosed and misdiagnosed. The semiologic discipline required here is to take subjective symptoms seriously and to map their quality—not just their presence.

6.1 Primary sensory cortex (postcentral gyrus)

Overview

Postcentral seizures most often begin with contralateral tingling or numbness, sometimes followed by a sensory march along the homunculus. Pain, heat, or other altered thermal sensations may also occur. In the large surgical series cited in the practical guide, contralateral somatosensory aura was the most common reported aura in parietal epilepsy.

Earliest and most localizing features

The most localizing onset clue is a unilateral distal contralateral somatosensory aura that is clearly restricted to a body region and especially if it marches in a somatotopic order. Marching sensory aura is one of the cleaner localizing signs in focal epilepsy and points strongly toward primary sensory cortex.

Usual propagation and semiologic evolution

As the seizure propagates to frontal motor cortex, the semiology may evolve into clonic motor activity or tonic posturing. This later motor phase can obscure the onset if the sensory component is not documented carefully.

Lateralizing implications

Unilateral sensory aura is usually contralateral to the side of onset. However, poorly localized whole-body sensations have little or no useful localizing value. The practical and classic reviews both insist on distinguishing orderly focal sensory symptoms from vague global sensations.

Main pitfalls and differential considerations

The main pitfall is failure to record the onset symptom because the sensory phase may be brief and subjective. Another is misclassifying painful or thermal sensations as non-epileptic if the clinician is unaware that parietal and posterior insular cortex can produce them.

6.2 Secondary sensory region and parietal operculum

Overview

The second somatosensory area and parietal opercular region can produce broader and less tidy somatosensory symptoms than primary sensory cortex. Sensations may involve distal extremities and the face and can be accompanied by a peculiar sense of inability to move the contralateral limbs. Heat or pain may also be prominent.

Earliest and most localizing features

The most localizing clue is a broad, often unpleasant somatosensory aura that is larger in territory than a simple postcentral march and may include the face or perioral region. A feeling of inability to move the contralateral limb in association with a sensory onset is especially useful.

Usual propagation and semiologic evolution

Spread from this region may recruit sensorimotor cortex, SMA, insula, or temporal structures, giving rise to clonic activity, tonic posturing, visceral symptoms, or automatisms.

Lateralizing implications

If the aura is unilateral, it is usually contralateral. However, because S2 and posterior insular symptoms may be bilateral or diffuse, the confidence of lateralization may be lower than for an orderly postcentral sensory march.

Main pitfalls and differential considerations

The main pitfall is confusion with posterior insular onset. In many cases the two can only be separated probabilistically from semiology, with invasive EEG needed for certainty.

6.3 Parietal association cortex and non-dominant body schema network

Figure 13. Upper part.

Figure 14. Autoscopic phenomena and vestibular networks.

Overview

Parietal association seizures are among the most distinctive but also the most easily dismissed. The non-dominant parietal association cortex can generate body image distortion, turning or twisting sensations, and altered body schema. Patients may describe a limb as enlarged, shrunken, absent, displaced, or transformed.

Earliest and most localizing features

The most localizing clues are qualitative distortions of body perception rather than simple tingling. Macrosomatognosis and microsomatognosis, particularly involving distal extremities, strongly suggest superior parietal or precuneal participation. Autoscopic phenomena and out-of-body-like experiences implicate a temporoparietal vestibular network rather than simple postcentral cortex (see figure below).

Figure 13. Illustrative semiology figure.

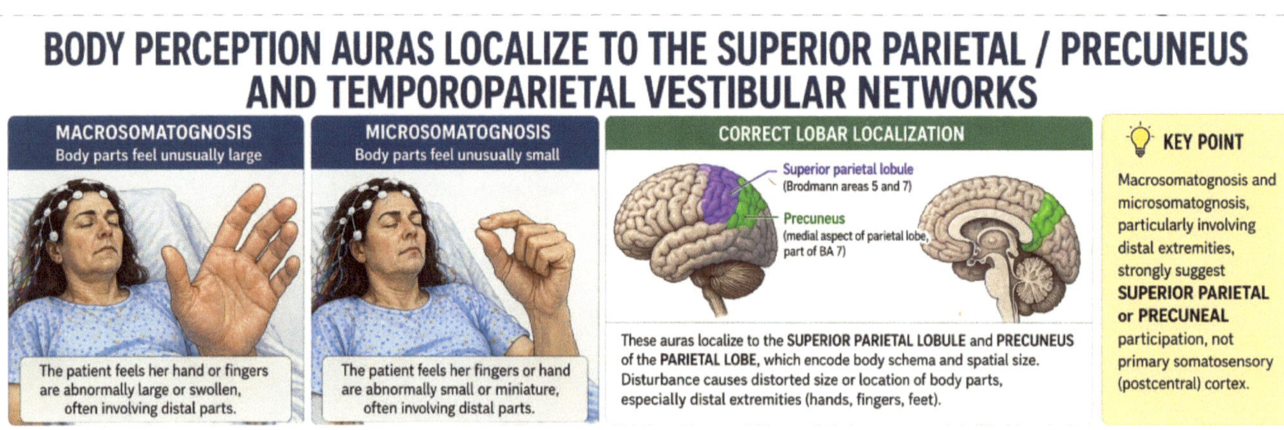

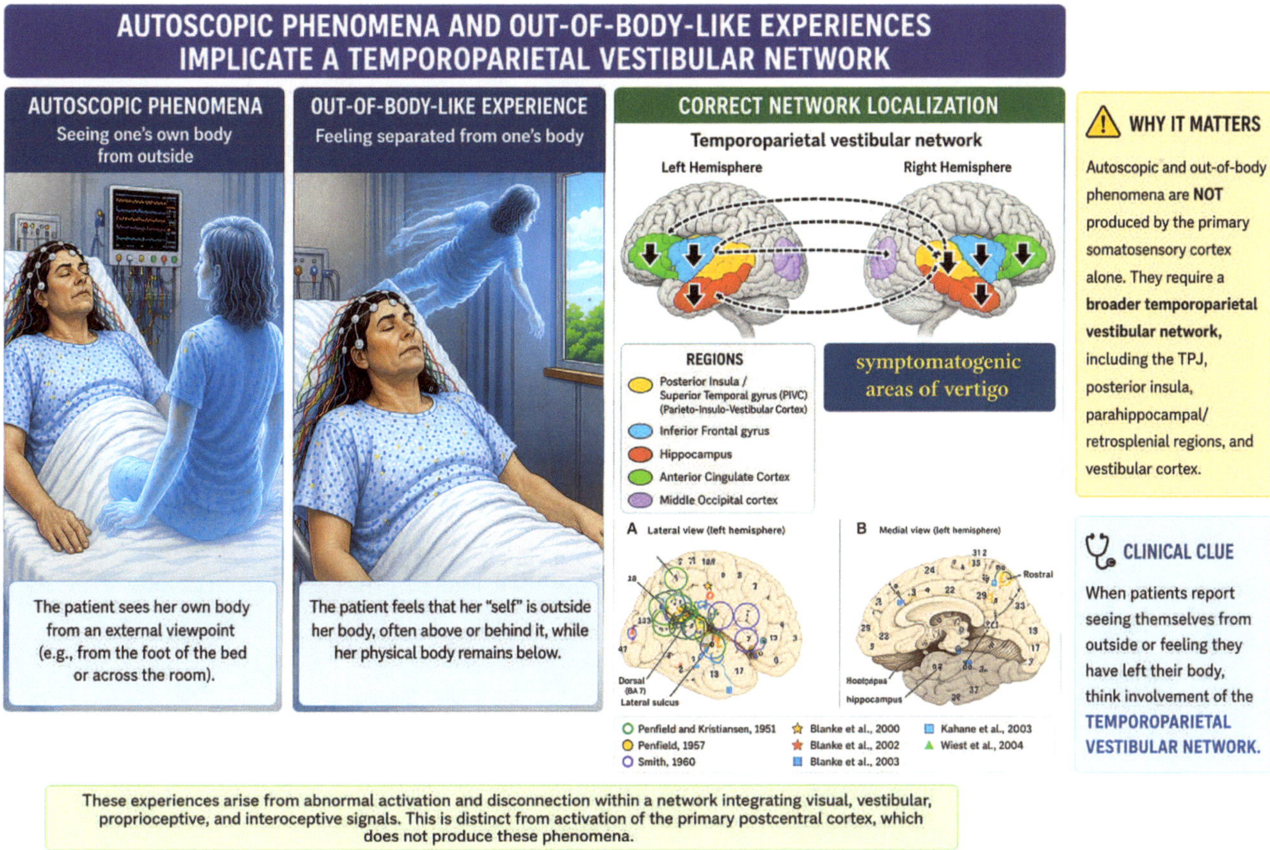

Usual propagation and semiologic evolution

These seizures frequently propagate into frontal or temporal networks. Once that happens, the semiology may acquire tonic posturing, clonic activity, or temporal aura/automatisms, which can mislead the observer away from the posterior onset.

Lateralizing implications

Lateralization from these symptoms is often difficult because body schema distortions are not always clearly lateralized in the patient narrative. If the symptom concerns one hemibody or one limb, the contralateral hemisphere is usually favored, but confidence is lower than for a simple sensory march or elementary visual aura.

Main pitfalls and differential considerations

The major pitfall is under-recognition. Patients may struggle to describe these experiences, and clinicians may not ask about them. Another pitfall is to call them 'psychic' or 'functional' rather than recognizing that they may be highly localizing to parietal association cortex.

6.4 Superior parietal lobule and intraparietal sulcus

Overview

The superior parietal lobule (SPL) and intraparietal sulcus participate in multisensory integration, body orientation, movement perception, and sensorimotor transformation. Seizures from this region are linked to altered body perception and to epileptic kinetopsia, the illusion that a stationary object is moving.

Earliest and most localizing features

The most useful onset signs are kinetopsia and higher-order body perception disturbance rather than simple numbness. In the reviewed literature the epileptic kinetopsia is localized to the superior parietal lobule and intraparietal sulcus.

Usual propagation and semiologic evolution

As spread occurs, seizures may recruit frontal motor or cingulate networks, producing tonic posturing, contralateral clonic activity, or a more concatenated semiology that looks frontal. Superior parietal seizures appear, in the practical guide, to spread preferentially to frontal areas.

Lateralizing implications

Lateralization is usually inferred from associated unilateral sensory or motor signs rather than from kinetopsia itself. If a contralateral limb distortion is clearly reported, it favors a focus in the opposite hemisphere.

Main pitfalls and differential considerations

The main pitfall is reducing these seizures to 'visual' or 'frontal' simply because the later semiology contains eye deviation or tonic posturing. The onset perceptual complaint carries more localizing weight than the later motor recruitment.

6.5 Precuneus

Overview

Precuneus seizures are increasingly recognized as a distinct subtype of medial parietal epilepsy. The precuneus is associated with altered visual perception, especially macropsia or micropsia. The dedicated systematic review on precuneus seizures adds that vestibular symptoms are the most common onset phenomenon, followed by visual illusions and body perception illusions; motor symptoms are more likely to emerge during propagation than at onset.

Earliest and most localizing features

The strongest localizing clues are vestibular onset, altered visual scale or self-location, and complex body perception disturbance, especially when the first subjective symptom is not a simple postcentral sensory aura or a classic temporal experiential aura. These symptoms should immediately prompt consideration of medial parietal onset.

Usual propagation and semiologic evolution

The precuneus is strongly connected to anterior frontal systems. There is a tendency for rapid anterior frontal spread, which helps explain why elementary or complex motor manifestations commonly appear later in the seizure and why some precuneus seizures are mistaken for frontal epilepsy.

Lateralizing implications

Lateralization is often challenging because vestibular and body-schema symptoms are not always experienced as clearly unilateral. When unilateral motor or sensory signs appear later, they follow the usual contralateral rule but should be recognized as propagated phenomena.

Main pitfalls and differential considerations

The main pitfall is frontal misclassification caused by rapid motorization of the seizure. Another is dismissing the initial vestibular or perceptual complaint as non-epileptic or migrainous. The review also stresses that the published literature on precuneus epilepsy remains sparse, which means that absence of a 'classic' pattern cannot exclude the diagnosis.

6.6 Inferior parietal lobule and temporoparietal junction (TPJ)

Overview

The inferior parietal and TPJ region sits at the intersection of vestibular, language, auditory, visual, and body-self processing. Seizures from this region may produce vertigo, autoscopy, altered self-location, reading/writing difficulty, and mixed perceptual experiences.

Earliest and most localizing features

The most localizing signs are autoscopic phenomena, vestibular-self disturbances, and dominant hemisphere reading/writing impairment early in the seizure. A mixture of visual, vestibular, and body-self disturbance is more suggestive of TPJ involvement than of a purely temporal or occipital focus.

Usual propagation and semiologic evolution

As spread reaches temporal areas, the seizure may acquire psychic aura or automatisms; if it reaches frontal systems, tonic or version-like motor signs may appear.

Lateralizing implications

Lateralization remains difficult unless the disturbance is clearly hemifield or hemibody specific or accompanied by unilateral motor/sensory signs. Dominant hemisphere language impairment at onset strongly suggests the dominant TPJ/perisylvian side.

Main pitfalls and differential considerations

The main pitfall is labeling autoscopy or vestibular symptoms as purely temporal because out-of-body-like experiences have long been associated with temporal lobe epilepsy. The literature reviewed explicitly reminds the reader that both temporal and parietal lobe epilepsies can generate autoscopic phenomena, with the TPJ and vestibular cortex acting as a shared network.

6.7 Painful parietal seizures

Overview

Pain as an ictal symptom is uncommon overall but clinically important because it is often overlooked or misinterpreted. Painful seizures are seen in 1.4% of monitored patients.

Earliest and most localizing features

The most localizing clue is a clearly ictal painful symptom—unilateral peripheral pain, cephalic pain, or abdominal pain—that occurs as an initial or early seizure manifestation rather than only postictally. In the painful seizure series, when the painful symptom was lateralized, it was contralateral to seizure onset.

Usual propagation and semiologic evolution

Painful parietal seizures may still evolve into more familiar sensory or motor patterns, but the early pain should not be dismissed. Some cases may be evaluated with invasive EEG because the clinical picture is unusual.

Lateralizing implications

Lateralization is contralateral when the pain is unilateral or clearly lateralized. Localization within the parietal network is less precise because painful symptoms may arise from different sensory territories and can overlap with posterior insular or secondary sensory cortex.

Main pitfalls and differential considerations

The main pitfall is diagnostic delay. Patients with isolated ictal pain may undergo extensive non-epileptic evaluation before epilepsy is considered. Another pitfall is misclassifying abdominal pain as temporal by default; the reviewed literature makes clear that abdominal pain can occur in parietal-onset seizures.

6.8 Parietal lobe synthesis

The parietal rule is that subjective phenomenology matters. A well-described onset complaint—distal numbness, thermal change, body-part enlargement, self-motion illusion, vestibular displacement, painful aura, inability to move despite preserved intention—often contains more localizing information than the later seizure video. Because parietal seizures spread in many directions, the observer must fight the urge to localize the event from its most visible late motor phase.

Clinical takeaway

- Best onset clue: focal sensory, body-schema, vestibular, or painful subjective onset.
- Best lateralizers: clearly unilateral sensory symptoms or later concordant motor asymmetry.
- Common trap: late tonic or hypermotor spread overcalled as mesial frontal onset.
- Escalate to invasive EEG when early subjective symptoms are subtle but consistently precede frontal-looking spread.

CHAPTER 7

Occipital Lobe Epilepsy

Occipital lobe seizures are most strongly associated with visual semiology, but the clinically visible seizure often reflects spread into temporal or frontal regions. Visual aura is common and often highly informative if the clinician characterizes it precisely: simple versus complex, hemifield versus diffuse, brief versus prolonged, and whether associated with eye deviation, blinking, or nystagmus.

7.1 Primary visual cortex (calcarine cortex)

Overview

The most classic occipital onset is an elementary visual aura from primary visual cortex. Patients may describe flashing bright lights, colored lights, or simple shapes, often spherical and brief. These phenomena are usually much shorter than migraine aura, commonly under two minutes.

Earliest and most localizing features

The most localizing onset pattern is a brief elementary visual aura, particularly when clearly lateralized to one hemifield. Both the practical guide and the classic review emphasize that hemifield visual aura has good lateralizing value to the contralateral occipital lobe.

Figure 15. Hemifield visual aura.

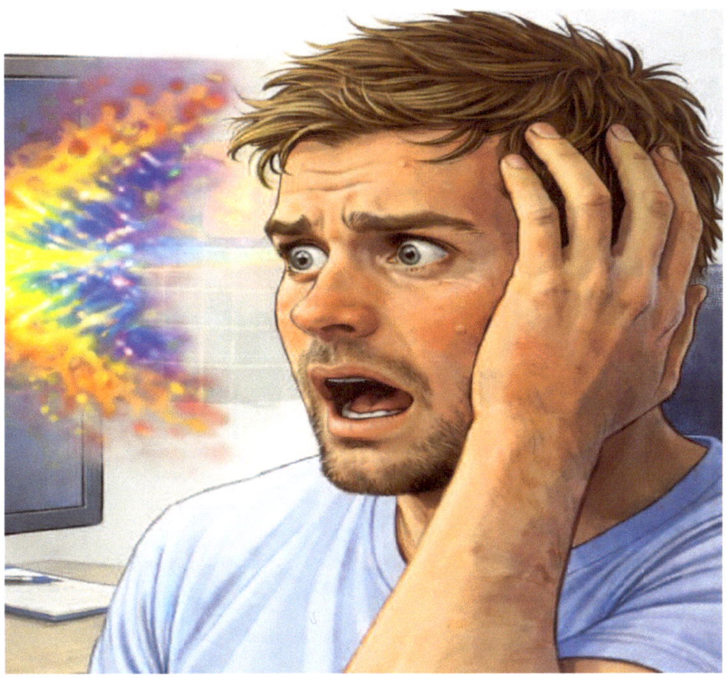

Figure. Right hemifield visual hallucination in a patient with left occipital epilepsy.

Usual propagation and semiologic evolution

As the discharge propagates, the seizure may acquire eye deviation, blinking, nystagmus, altered awareness, or later temporal/frontal features. The primary visual aura therefore has to be captured before the later spread obscures the onset.

Lateralizing implications

Hemifield elementary visual symptoms lateralize contralaterally. Up to around one-third of patients, however, may experience more diffuse or poorly lateralized visual change, reducing confidence in side assignment.

Main pitfalls and differential considerations

The main pitfall is confusion with migraine. OLE is often misdiagnosed as having migraine visual aura. The practical distinction is that epileptic visual aura is usually brief, stereotyped, and often followed by further ictal evolution, whereas migraine aura tends to be longer and followed by headache rather than an epileptic motor sequence.

7.2 Visual association cortex and prestriate occipital regions

Overview

When seizures involve visual association cortex rather than primary visual cortex, the visual experience becomes more complex: formed hallucinations, visual scene fragments, kinetopsia, macropsia, micropsia, or rarely autoscopy. These symptoms may still reflect occipital onset but often imply spread into temporo-parietal association networks.

Earliest and most localizing features

The strongest localizing clue is a complex visual perceptual distortion appearing at onset, especially when it is repetitive and stereotyped across seizures. Kinetopsia and size distortion are particularly useful because they tie the seizure to higher-order visual association cortex rather than to mesial temporal experiential aura alone.

Usual propagation and semiologic evolution

These seizures often propagate into temporal lobe, generating automatisms or psychic phenomena, or into parietal cortex, generating more extensive spatial or body-perception disturbance.

Lateralizing implications

Lateralization is less secure than with hemifield elementary visual aura unless the phenomenon is clearly restricted to one hemifield or paired with unilateral motor signs. Still, complex visual onset remains strongly localizing to a posterior visual network.

Main pitfalls and differential considerations

The main pitfall is to label all complex hallucinations as temporal. The practical guide explicitly notes that complex visual hallucinations may occur in occipital epilepsy when the prestriate cortex is involved or when the seizure spreads into adjacent temporo-parietal regions.

7.3 Parieto-occipital junction

Overview

The parieto-occipital junction is particularly associated with oculomotor semiology: eye deviation, blinking, and epileptic nystagmus. This region should be considered whenever the first visible sign is ocular but the history suggests a posterior sensory onset.

Earliest and most localizing features

The most useful localizing clues are early eye deviation, blinking, or nystagmus occurring in close proximity to a visual aura or even as the onset itself. The practical guide notes that in a large series approximately one-fifth of patients had eye blinking at seizure onset, and that epileptic nystagmus usually has its fast phase directed contralaterally.

Usual propagation and semiologic evolution

If the seizure progresses, temporal or frontal semiology may quickly emerge. Thus, an event that appears to begin with eye version should still be reviewed for a preceding subjective visual symptom.

Lateralizing implications

Unilateral eye blinking lateralizes ipsilaterally, whereas the fast phase of epileptic nystagmus points contralaterally. These are useful but must be distinguished from nonspecific eyelid flutter or nonversive ocular movements.

Main pitfalls and differential considerations

The main pitfall is overcalling frontal eye field onset simply because version is present. Posterior seizures can produce ocular manifestations, and the timing relative to visual aura matters greatly.

7.4 Mesial versus lateral occipital considerations

Overview

Occipital epilepsy is clinically heterogeneous and that mesial versus lateral occipital onset may differ in electroclinical patterns, although the bedside distinction is not always easy. Mesial occipital seizures may be especially prone to stereotyped visual aura, whereas lateral occipital or border-zone seizures may more readily acquire pulsating or more elaborate perceptual qualities.

Earliest and most localizing features

The earliest visual phenomenon remains more useful than the mesial-lateral label itself. A brief, stereotyped, elementary, hemifield visual aura should keep the focus on primary occipital onset regardless of later spread.

Usual propagation and semiologic evolution

Propagated temporal or frontal semiology is common, especially in long seizures or in cases that secondarily generalize.

Lateralizing implications

Lateralization remains stronger than sublobar localization in many occipital cases. Hemifield aura, nystagmus fast phase, and concordant later unilateral motor signs help more than the exact shape or color of the visual phenomenon alone.

Main pitfalls and differential considerations

The pitfall is false certainty. Although certain visual qualities have been linked historically to lateral versus mesial occipital onset, the literature does not support rigid overuse of those distinctions without invasive or imaging correlation.

7.5 Occipital lobe synthesis

For occipital epilepsy, precision of history is everything. The clinician should ask about color, brightness, motion, shape, hemifield, duration, and whether the symptom is positive or negative. A two-sentence careful aura history often localizes the seizure better than a full description of the later bilateral tonic-clonic phase.

Clinical takeaway

- Best onset clue: a precisely characterized elementary or complex visual aura.
- Best lateralizers: hemifield visual symptoms, with ocular signs interpreted cautiously and in sequence.
- Common trap: migraine or late temporal/frontal spread obscuring a posterior onset.
- Escalate to invasive EEG when parieto-occipital overlap or complex visual semiology blurs boundaries.

CHAPTER 8

Cingulate Network Epilepsy

The cingulate cortex is best understood as an anterior-posterior gradient with markedly different clinical implications. Anterior cingulate seizures more often generate emotional-autonomic and hypermotor syndromes, whereas posterior cingulate seizures frequently mimic temporal or extratemporal epilepsy and only reveal their identity when propagation patterns are analyzed carefully or invasive EEG is performed.

8.1 Anterior cingulate cortex

Overview

Anterior cingulate seizures are characterized by intense fright, screaming, vocalization, autonomic activation, complex gestural automatisms, and hypermotor activity. Some cases instead show simpler motor phenomena with more frequent generalization, especially in lesional disease.

Earliest and most localizing features

The earliest localizing clue is a combination of fear or alarm-like affect with vocalization, autonomic activation, and early hypermotor or gestural behavior.

Figure 16. Anterior cingulate seizure in progress.

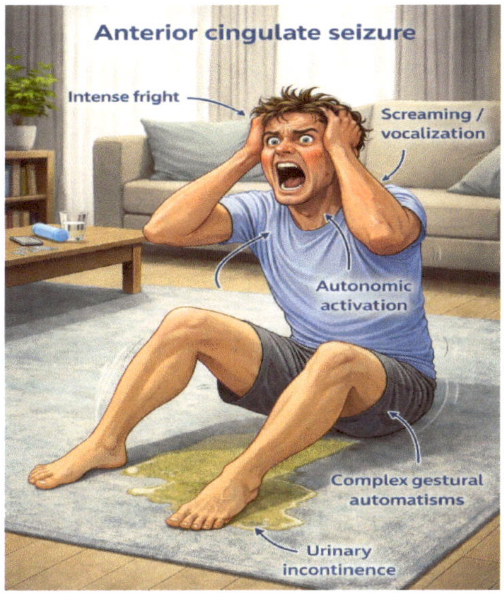

Hypermotor behavior, autonomic symptoms, and fear during an anterior cingulate seizure.

If an ictal pout appears early, anterior cingulate or nearby mesiofrontal involvement becomes even more likely.

Figure 17. Seizure semiology anterior cingulate seizure.

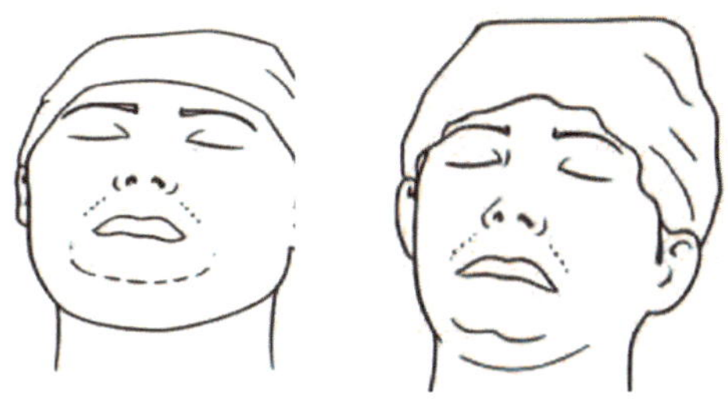

Chapeau de gendarme Sign.

Usual propagation and semiologic evolution

These seizures often spread quickly into broader frontal motor networks, producing bilateral asymmetric tonic or complex hypermotor patterns. Because of this, the seizure may appear purely frontal unless the early emotional-autonomic phase is documented.

Lateralizing implications

Lateralization usually depends on accompanying unilateral motor signs. The fear or scream itself has little reliable side value.

Main pitfalls and differential considerations

The main pitfall is mistaking anterior cingulate fear for mesial temporal fear. Anterior cingulate fear is usually embedded in a motor-autonomic storm rather than in a quieter experiential aura followed by classic temporal automatisms.

Figure 19. Anterior cingulate seizures with fear vs mesial temporal seizure with fear

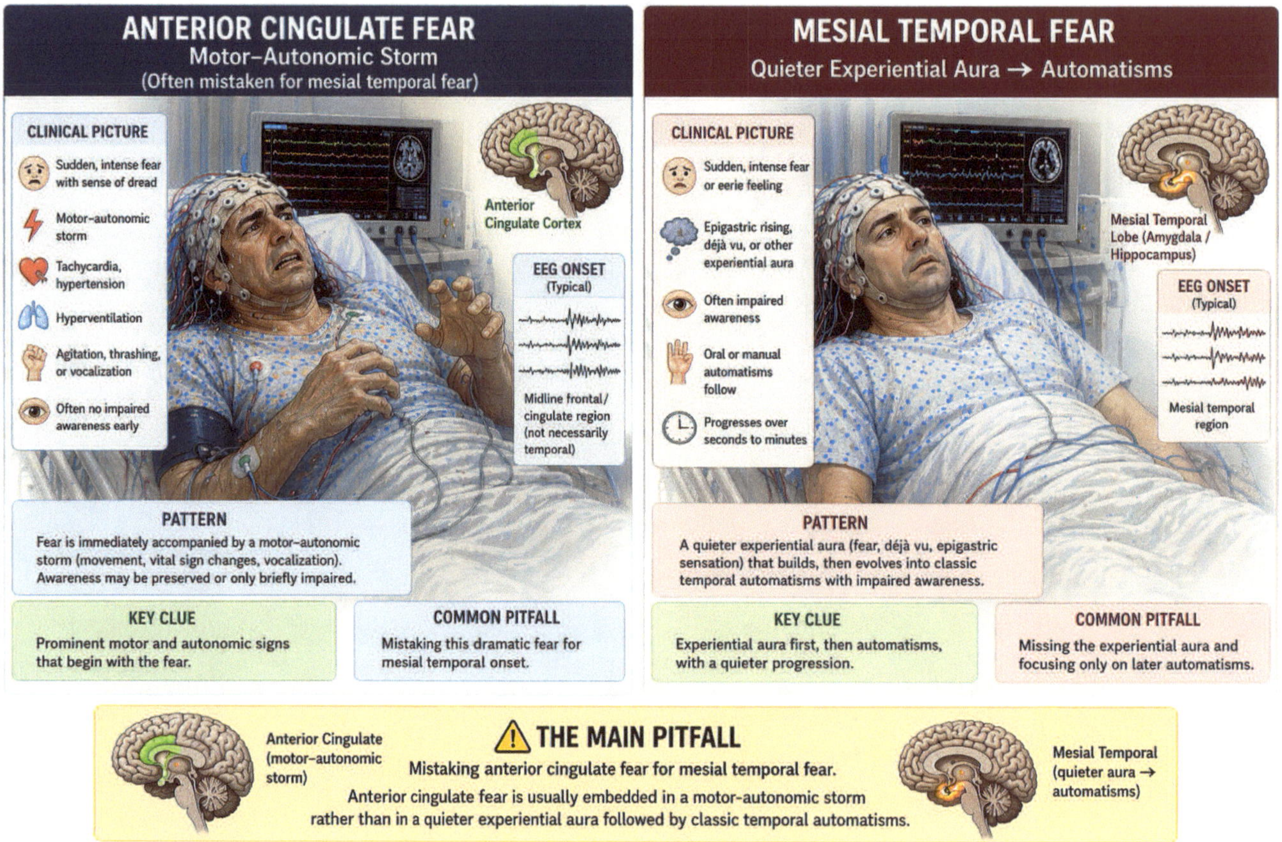

8.2 Posterior cingulate cortex (general principles)

Overview

Posterior cingulate epilepsy is uncommon but clinically important because it closely mimics both temporal and extratemporal epilepsies. An SEEG study of 15 patients and 59 seizures emphasizes that behavioral arrest is the dominant manifestation across posterior cingulate subregions and that scalp EEG often has limited localizing power because the cortex is deep and relatively clinically silent until spread occurs.

Earliest and most localizing features

The earliest and most useful clues are often subtle: dizziness, vertigo, visual blurring, déjà vu, jamais vu, rising epigastric sensation, autonomic symptoms, or an early dialeptic pause before more expressive temporal or frontal semiology emerges. The posterior cingulate should be considered when the seizure looks 'temporal' but the anatomy and invasive data do not fit, especially when symptoms are vestibular or polymorphic.

Usual propagation and semiologic evolution

Propagation pattern is the real key. When posterior cingulate discharges spread to temporal structures, the seizure often looks dialeptic or automotor. When they spread to frontal or mesial frontal regions, the seizure may become bilateral asymmetric tonic or hypermotor. Some cases develop axial tonic seizures when spread reaches midcingulate, precentral, or precuneal networks.

Lateralizing implications

Lateralization from posterior cingulate semiology alone is usually limited. Associated unilateral motor signs retain their usual value, but the posterior cingulate syndrome itself is more localizing by network suspicion than by side certainty.

Main pitfalls and differential considerations

The main pitfall is temporal misclassification. The uploaded SEEG paper repeatedly shows that posterior cingulate seizures can present with behavioral arrest, automatisms, psychic aura, abdominal aura, or gustatory phenomena because temporal spread occurs quickly.

8.3 Dorsal posterior cingulate cortex (dPCC)

Overview

The dorsal posterior cingulate appears to have stronger frontal and vestibular associations than the ventral sector. In the uploaded SEEG and stimulation data, vestibular responses were especially common in dPCC and retrosplenial cortex.

Earliest and most localizing features

The most localizing early clues are dizziness or vertigo, especially when accompanied by other posterior self-motion or visuospatial symptoms. Pure clinical seizures directly elicited from this cortex were rare, underscoring how often the clinically visible seizure reflects spread rather than isolated dPCC symptomatogenic activation.

Usual propagation and semiologic evolution

As seizures propagate to frontal or motor networks, the clinical picture may acquire axial tonic, neck, or upper-limb motor features. This is particularly relevant when dPCC involvement spreads toward midcingulate and premotor systems.

Lateralizing implications

Lateralization is usually poor unless vestibular symptoms are clearly lateralized or accompanied by unilateral motor signs. The stimulation study suggested a predominance of vestibular responses in the left hemisphere, but this is not yet a bedside lateralizing rule that should be overused clinically.

Main pitfalls and differential considerations

The main pitfall is to dismiss dizziness or visual blurring as nonspecific. In a patient with otherwise unexplained polymorphic focal seizures, these symptoms should prompt consideration of posterior cingulate or medial parietal cortex.

8.4 Ventral posterior cingulate cortex (vPCC)

Overview

The ventral posterior cingulate is more tightly linked to temporal structures than the dorsal sector. When ictal activity extended to mesial and lateral temporal cortex, automatisms were predominantly observed in seizures originating from the ventral PCC. Behavioral arrest and autonomic symptoms were also common.

Earliest and most localizing features

The most localizing onset clues are behavioral arrest with early autonomic symptoms such as palpitations, tachycardia, nausea, or epigastric discomfort, especially when the later seizure becomes automotor and temporal-like. This combination is a classic setting in which ventral PCC should be in the hypothesis set.

Usual propagation and semiologic evolution

The usual evolution is rapid spread to hippocampus and other temporal structures, which can produce oral and gestural automatisms, later dystonic posture, and longer dialeptic phases. In the uploaded series, some ventral PCC cases reached bilateral or ipsilateral hippocampus within 0–1 second.

Lateralizing implications

Lateralization again is modest from syndrome alone and is better inferred from the associated unilateral dystonia, tonic asymmetry, or other lateralizing signs during spread.

Main pitfalls and differential considerations

The main pitfall is false mesial temporal localization. When a seizure begins with epigastric sensation or déjà vu and then becomes automotor, ventral PCC is not the first bedside hypothesis, yet the uploaded invasive data show that it can generate exactly this pattern through extremely rapid temporal recruitment.

8.5 Retrosplenial cortex (RSC)

Overview

The retrosplenial cortex has the strongest relationship in the uploaded set to complex motor behavior and visual/vestibular responses. SEEG studies. have found that RSC-origin seizures often evolved into integrated complex motor behavior while spreading to hippocampal and temporal structures. Stimulation of the RSC also elicited the largest number of visual responses.

Earliest and most localizing features

The most localizing clues are a posterior self-motion or visual disturbance followed by integrated complex motor behavior that still feels more 'posterior-temporal' than classical frontal hypermotor epilepsy. Longer impairment of consciousness was also noted in the RSC group compared with the vPCC group.

Usual propagation and semiologic evolution

Propagation commonly reaches hippocampus, temporal pole, long insular gyrus, or posterior temporal neocortex, which explains why the final seizure may look automotor or temporal. Axial or limb tonic manifestations may also appear if mesial frontal or midcingulate regions are recruited.

Lateralizing implications

Lateralization from RSC syndrome alone is limited. Visual symptoms may help if clearly lateralized, but many RSC phenomena are more network-level than hemifield-specific.

Main pitfalls and differential considerations

The main pitfall is to interpret the late complex motor behavior as proof of frontal onset. In the uploaded data, those complex behaviors could arise from RSC onset with subsequent temporal spread.

8.6 Cingulate network synthesis

The cingulate lesson is that propagation pattern is often more informative than the final seizure phenotype. Anterior cingulate tends to declare itself through affective-autonomic-hypermotor onset. Posterior cingulate, especially ventral PCC and retrosplenial cortex, often borrows the clinical language of temporal epilepsy and must be recognized by its subtle posterior clues and by the mismatch between bedside temporal semiology and invasive anatomical truth.

Clinical takeaway

- Best onset clue: affective-autonomic-hypermotor onset for anterior cingulate, subtle posterior self-motion symptoms for posterior cingulate.
- Best lateralizers: accompanying unilateral motor signs rather than emotion, fear, or automatisms alone.
- Common trap: temporal or frontal mimicry created by rapid propagation.
- Escalate to invasive EEG when deep cingulate onset is plausible and scalp EEG is nonlocalizing.

CHAPTER 9

Special Network-Linked Seizures and High-Yield Syndrome Clues

9.1 Gelastic seizures and hypothalamic hamartoma

Overview

Gelastic seizures most classically arise from hypothalamic hamartoma and usually begin in early childhood. They are typically brief, stereotyped, frequent, often mirthless, and may occur without clear impairment of consciousness, though autonomic signs such as flushing and pupillary dilation are common.

Earliest and most localizing features

The most localizing clue is age plus pattern: very early childhood onset, frequent brief mirthless laughter, and stereotypy strongly support hypothalamic hamartoma. Adult-onset gelastic seizures are less likely to be hypothalamic and may instead arise from temporal or frontal networks.

Usual propagation and semiologic evolution

When the source is outside the hypothalamus, the laughter is usually one component of a more complex seizure that may include automotor features or altered awareness.

Lateralizing implications

Lateralization is generally weak; localization depends more on syndrome and imaging than on side-specific semiology.

Main pitfalls and differential considerations

The pitfall is overlocalizing laughter to one region. The practical approach is to consider that laughter belongs to a broader network including cingulate, frontal, and temporal regions.

9.2 Chapeau de gendarme (ictal pout)

Overview

Ictal pouting or chapeau de gendarme refers to a downturned mouth produced by bilateral contraction of the lips and chin. If sign occurs early, it is highly localizing to frontal lobe onset, especially anterior cingulate, orbitofrontal, mesioprefrontal, or premotor regions.

Earliest and most localizing features

The most localizing use of the sign is early occurrence. If the pout appears after a complex hypermotor sequence has already developed, it is less specific than if it appears among the first visible objective signs.

Usual propagation and semiologic evolution

The sign may coexist with rocking, chewing, head movement, or other frontal motor behavior as the seizure evolves.

Lateralizing implications

The sign has more localizing than lateralizing value; side assignment comes from accompanying unilateral signs.

Main pitfalls and differential considerations

The main pitfall is late overinterpretation. In practice, the same facial movement may occur later in seizures that did not begin in the frontal lobe. Timing is everything.

9.3 Reflex seizures with localizing value

Overview

Reflex seizures are not a lobe, but some reflex triggers carry useful localizing implications. For instance, photosensitive focal epilepsy suggests occipital onset; musicogenic seizures localize to the temporal lobe; startle-induced tonic or atonic seizures suggest onset in or near the supplementary motor area; and eating-induced seizures usually arise from temporal or extratemporal perisylvian regions.

Earliest and most localizing features

The earliest localizing clue is the specific trigger itself, but only when the trigger is reproducible and the event is truly epileptic rather than behavioral or nonepileptic.

Usual propagation and semiologic evolution

As with spontaneous seizures, propagation may then recruit wider networks and produce semiology that no longer looks reflex-specific.

Lateralizing implications

Lateralization depends on the later semiology, not on the trigger alone.

Main pitfalls and differential considerations

The main pitfall is overconfidence from the trigger without confirmation that the event is electroclinical epilepsy. Reflex triggers are useful only when the diagnosis is secure.

Clinical takeaway

- Best onset clue: define the syndrome first and then reconstruct its sequence.
- Best lateralizers: derive from accompanying unilateral motor or language signs, not from the syndrome label alone.
- Common trap: overlocalizing from a dramatic trigger, gelastic laughter, or ictal pout without chronology.
- Escalate to invasive EEG when syndrome and imaging do not match or when network spread dominates the bedside picture.

CHAPTER 10

Cross-Cutting Ictal Lateralizing Signs

Some signs lateralize much better than they localize. These high-yield bedside markers are clinically valuable because they remain useful even when lobe localization is uncertain. The literature consistently emphasize that the strongest lateralizing signs are often motor or postictal rather than experiential.

Top bedside lateralizers at a glance

Early true version, figure-of-four, unilateral dystonia, unilateral focal clonus, the last clonic jerk, postictal aphasia, and contextual postictal nosewiping are among the highest-yield side markers when they are timed correctly and defined strictly.

10.1 High-yield lateralizing sign matrix

Sign	Typical side rule	Localization value	Main cautions
Early true version	Contralateral to seizure onset	Low-to-moderate (improved by latency analysis)	Must distinguish from nonversive turning; can occur in frontal and extrafrontal epilepsy
Figure-of-four posture	Extended arm is contralateral to seizure onset	Poor lobe localization	Best used near secondary generalization
Fencing posture / M2e pattern	Raised/extended arm contralateral	Suggests SMA recruitment, not necessarily SMA onset	May reflect spread from parietal/occipital onset
Unilateral dystonic posturing	Contralateral to seizure onset	Limited lobe localization; common in TLE	Often requires adequate duration and clarity
Unilateral clonic onset	Contralateral to seizure onset	Good when onset is early and focal	Later clonus may reflect spread

Sign	Typical side rule	Localization value	Main cautions
Last clonic jerk	Ipsilateral to seizure onset	No lobe localization	Most useful in focal-to-bilateral tonic-clonic seizures
Todd paresis	Contralateral to seizure onset	Not localizing	Must be true postictal weakness
Unilateral eye blinking	Ipsilateral to seizure onset	Low localization	Differentiate from flutter or nonspecific blinking
Epileptic nystagmus fast phase	Contralateral to seizure onset	Suggests occipital or temporo-occipital network	Rare; requires careful ocular analysis
Preserved awareness during temporal automatisms	Supports non-dominant hemisphere	Applies mainly in temporal epilepsy	Not absolute
Ictal/postictal dysphasia	Supports dominant hemisphere	Poor lobe localization	Differentiate from speech arrest
RINCH motions	Contralateral in temporal lobe epilepsy	Temporal context needed	Not universal

10.2 Version, timing, and head position evolution

Version is one of the most useful ictal lateralizing signs in focal epilepsy, but only when defined strictly. Tufenkjian & Lüders and the 2025 timing study both insist that version must be forced, sustained, unnatural, and accompanied by a characteristic upward-turned chin and head posture. Natural appearing head turning or scanning eye movements have much weaker value.

The 2025 study by Sivaji et al. adds an underused nuance: latency from seizure onset to version carries localizing information. Frontal seizures reached version earliest, temporal seizures later, and occipital seizures latest. A seizure with true version within 15 seconds should strongly raise frontal lobe onset in the differential. This does not mean all later version is nonlocalizing; it means late version is more likely to reflect spread to the frontal eye field.

A second important finding from the same study is that in a subset of secondarily generalized seizures the head evolved from initial version to a midline position and then to a late ictal-end position opposite the initial version. This late ictal-end head position was always ipsilateral to the epileptogenic zone in that subset. Although this is not a first-line sign, it is clinically valuable when reviewing focal-to-bilateral tonic-clonic seizures frame by frame.

Evidence highlight

A complementary spontaneous-seizure cohort by Fotedar et al. (2022) adds useful bedside granularity to what true version looks like. In 43 versive seizures, eye movements were conjugate in all seizures and contralateral in 100% of clearly focal lateralized onsets. The eyes were usually saccadic rather than smooth (89.3%) and most often had an oblique upward vector rather than a purely horizontal one. Head deviation accompanied eye deviation in all seizures, moved in the same direction in 97.6%, and commonly showed an upward chin component, while ipsilateral tonic-clonic facial motor activity accompanied version in 93%. Practically, forced oblique upward gaze with coupled head turning and ipsilateral facial recruitment remains entirely compatible with frontal eye field version and should not be dismissed as a nonspecific motor phenomenon.

10.3 Figure-of-four, fencing, tonic asymmetry, and clonic ending

The figure-of-four sign and the fencing posture remain indispensable in convulsive semiology review. The extended arm points contralaterally to seizure onset. A fencing posture early in a brief mesial frontal seizure strongly suggests SMA recruitment and may reflect onset there. The same posture appearing after a parietal sensory onset likely reflects spread to SMA rather than primary mesial frontal epilepsy.

Similarly, the last clonic jerk of a bilateral tonic-clonic seizure is usually ipsilateral to the side of onset, and Todd paresis is usually contralateral. These are powerful side markers but poor sublobar localizers.

10.4 Language and dominance-related signs

Ictal or postictal dysphasia lateralizes to the dominant hemisphere but does not reliably distinguish frontal from temporal dominant-side recruitment. Ictal speech with meaningful or at least intelligible verbalization during impaired awareness tends to support the non-dominant hemisphere, especially in temporal lobe epilepsy, though exceptions occur often enough that this should be treated as supportive rather than definitive.

Speech arrest and aphasic impairment must be differentiated. Speech arrest can arise from frontal motor or language-blocking mechanisms and is not a lateralizing sign by itself. Aphasia with preserved engagement but impaired naming, repetition, reading, or comprehension is more anatomically informative.

10.5 Autonomic and non-dominant temporal indicators

Peri-ictal drinking, ictal spitting, ictal vomiting, and an urge to urinate are repeatedly described as markers favoring a non-dominant temporal focus. They are useful because they can provide side information in otherwise bilateral-looking temporal seizures.

These signs have relatively poor lobe specificity outside the temporal context and should therefore be used within an already plausible temporal syndrome rather than as free-standing localizers.

Evidence highlight

Another underused temporal side marker is postictal nosewiping. In a blinded video review of 87 patients and 319 non-generalized complex partial seizures, Hirsch et al. (1998) found that postictal nosewiping within 60 seconds of EEG offset was more common in unilateral temporal than extratemporal epilepsy, and when a patient with temporal lobe epilepsy wiped the nose with one hand only, the wiping hand was ipsilateral to seizure onset in 92% of cases. Repetitive same-hand postictal nosewiping within a single seizure was ipsilateral in all recorded temporal cases. The sign should still be interpreted as supportive rather than decisive, because extratemporal seizures can occasionally show similar behavior, but in an otherwise plausible temporal syndrome it compares favorably with many classic postictal lateralizers.

10.6 Hand postures

Figure 20. Figure. Hand postures in patients with frontal, temporal, and generalized epilepsy.

I) I) Patient with left temporal lobe sclerosis.

II) Patient with right frontal lobe epilepsy.

III) Patient with generalized tonic-clonic seizure.

IV) Patient with left temporal lobe epilepsy.

V) Patient with right frontal lobe epilepsy.

VI) Patient with left temporal lobe epilepsy.

Figure 20. Hand posturing in seizures: Localizing value.

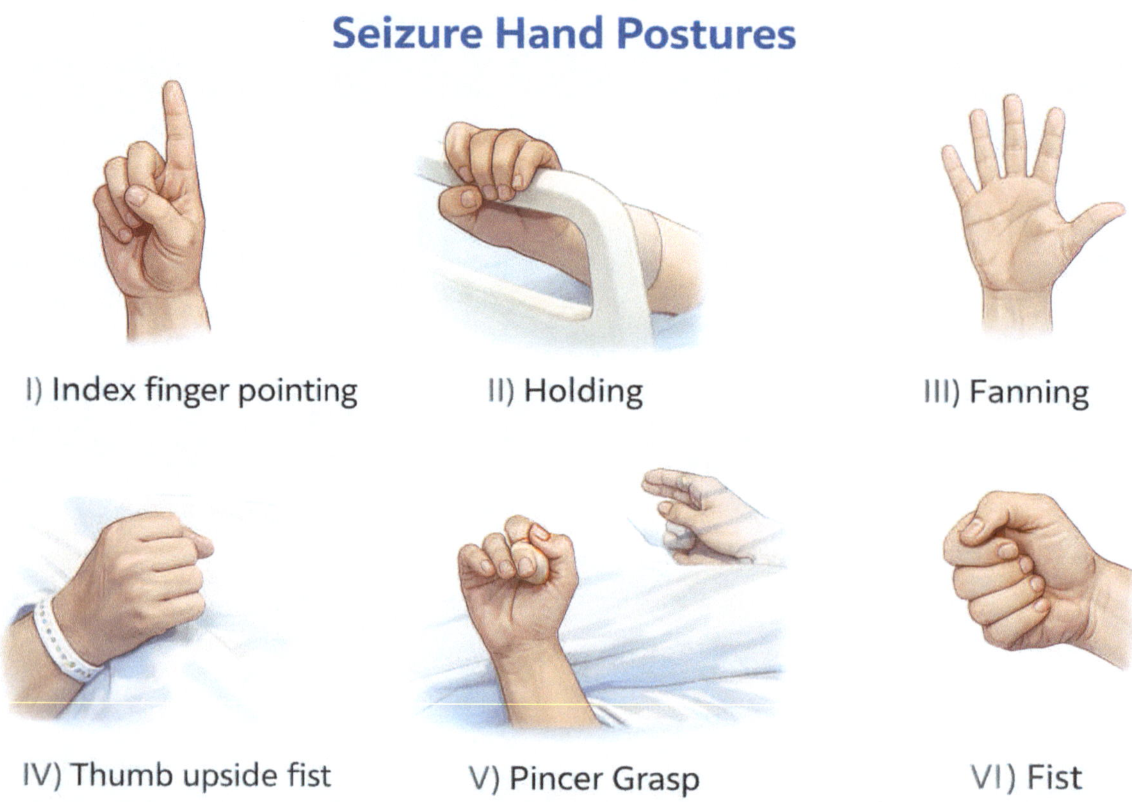

Pediatric note

The pediatric hand posture cohort adds an important modern bedside layer to classic lateralization. In that study, fist posture was most frequent in frontal lobe seizures, thumb-upside fist was more typical of temporal lobe seizures, and fanning posture was most common in generalized seizures. Ipsilateral hand posture was more common in frontal lobe seizures, whereas contralateral hand posture was more common in temporal lobe seizures. These findings are promising because they are simple to annotate from family video and from video-EEG, but they still require validation with broader invasive or postsurgical correlation.

Clinical takeaway

- Best use: treat hand posture as a supportive, age-aware side clue rather than a stand-alone localizer.
- Best current pattern: fist posture favored frontal seizures, thumb-upside fist favored temporal seizures, and fanning favored generalized seizures in the reviewed pediatric cohort.

- Common trap: applying pediatric motor-expression rules directly to adults or overcalling lobe localization from posture alone.
- Escalate to broader multimodal correlation whenever hand posture conflicts with earlier aura or first visible sign.

Hand posture	Most associated setting in uploaded paper	Side tendency	Interpretive note
Fist	Frontal lobe seizures in children	Often ipsilateral	Useful adjunct, not stand-alone
Thumb-upside fist	Temporal lobe seizures in children	Often contralateral	May be especially helpful when combined with other temporal signs
Fanning	Generalized seizures	Not a focal lateralizing sign	Can help prevent false focal labeling
Index-finger pointing / pincer grasp	Reported but less established	Not yet reliable	Age and rapid spread may modify appearance
Ictal grasping	Most characteristic of frontal hyperkinetic seizures	No reliable lateralizing value	May be occasional purposeful movement in extrafrontal seizures

CHAPTER 11

Practical Differential Diagnosis by Sequence Pattern

11.1 Frontal versus temporal

Feature	Frontal tendency	Temporal tendency	Practical weight
Onset	Abrupt	More gradual	Moderate
Duration	Usually brief	Often longer	Moderate
Sleep predominance	Common	Less common	Supportive
Automatisms	Less common and shorter	More common and longer	Moderate
Complex motor/hypermotor	Early and prominent	Later and less frequent except temporal pole/plus	Moderate
Postictal confusion	Shorter	Longer	Moderate
Aura	Often absent or short	Common and informative	High if well described
Version timing	Earlier	Later	Helpful if

Feature	Frontal tendency	Temporal tendency	Practical weight
			documented

This matrix should not be read as a checklist where the highest count wins. Rather, it is a sequence tool: an epigastric rising sensation followed by oral automatisms and later version still favors mesial temporal onset even if the seizure becomes strongly motor. By contrast, a brief sleep-related seizure that begins with abrupt bilateral asymmetric tonic posturing and no meaningful aura still favors SMA or another frontal network even if awareness is lost immediately thereafter.

A quantitative SEEG-based analysis of 55 hyperkinetic seizures further explains why bedside hypermotor behavior resists a simple frontal-versus-temporal dichotomy. Fayerstein et al. (2020) found that bilateral symmetric stereotyped hyperkinesia without dystonia mapped to a mixed temporal and dorsolateral prefrontal pattern, whereas emotionally colored, vocal, integrated bilateral hyperkinesia clustered with ventromedial prefrontal seizures but still occurred in roughly half of temporal hyperkinetic seizures. Just as importantly, asymmetric or unilateral hyperkinetic movement with marked dystonia and a clearer aura favored parietal onset rather than frontal onset. The practical implication is that hyperkinetic seizures should be subdivided by symmetry, dystonia, emotionality, integrated behavior, and aura timing before assigning a frontal label.

11.2 Temporal versus temporal-plus

Evidence highlight

The most clinically important distinction is that visual hallucinations and vertigo should raise suspicion for temporal-plus epilepsy rather than conventional temporal lobe epilepsy. In contrast, early manual and oral automatisms, late dystonic posture, and late head version fit more comfortably within conventional temporal lobe seizures. In practice, this means that posterior sensory aura should not be 'explained away' by later temporal automatisms.

11.3 Parietal versus occipital versus insular sensory onset

A helpful bedside separation is to ask whether the earliest symptom is primarily somatosensory, visual, or visceral-autonomic. A focal distal marching paresthesia favors postcentral cortex. A broad painful or bilateral sensory dysesthesia favors posterior insula or S2/opercular participation. A brief elementary visual aura favors primary visual cortex. Complex body-schema distortion or vestibular-self disturbance suggests parietal association, TPJ, or precuneus. Visceral-laryngeal-autonomic onset with broad somatic discomfort favors anterior insula.

11.4 Cingulate versus frontal versus temporal mimicry

Anterior cingulate seizures can mimic frontal hypermotor epilepsy; posterior cingulate seizures can mimic temporal automotor epilepsy. The practical discriminator is often the earliest emotional-autonomic sign for anterior cingulate and the subtle posterior perceptual or vestibular clue for posterior cingulate.

Clinical takeaway

- First question: what happened first?
- Highest-yield separations: frontal versus temporal, temporal versus temporal-plus, sensory-onset distinctions, and cingulate mimics.

- Common trap: anchoring on late motor spectacle instead of early sensory or experiential onset.
- Escalate to invasive EEG when the semiology is hybrid or multimodal data remain discordant.

CHAPTER 12

Limitations of Lateralization and Localization Analysis in Epilepsy

The literature is unusually consistent in one respect: seizure semiology is indispensable, but it is not self-sufficient. Tufenkjian & Lüders state this most directly by identifying the main limitations of semiology as a localizing tool. First, semiology is subjective. Even highly trained epileptologists show inter-rater variability, especially when distinguishing versive from nonversive head turning, deciding whether a movement is dystonic or tonic, or deciding whether a behavior is purposeful, hypermotor, or automotor. Standardization helps, but it does not abolish disagreement.

Second, semiology reflects the symptomatogenic zone rather than automatically revealing the seizure-onset zone or epileptogenic zone. This is the most important limitation. The same symptom can be produced when seizures from different origins recruit the same eloquent cortex; conversely, seizures beginning in the same region can produce different symptoms depending on state, spread pattern, and network engagement. This principle is not a theoretical caveat—it is exactly why parietal, insular, orbitofrontal, posterior cingulate, and precuneus epilepsies are so easily mislocalized from bedside appearance alone.

Third, the localizing value of a sign depends heavily on its timing. Late signs may only show spread. If a clinician extracts a semiology list without a timeline, the result may be internally contradictory and anatomically misleading. The clinical solution is not to discard semiology, but to reconstruct seizure time carefully and weight the earliest and most specific events most strongly.

Fourth, scalp EEG and semiology are not interchangeable. Chowdhury et al. remind the reader that EEG electrodes detect ictal recruitment and input, not necessarily the exact cortical site generating the observed behavior. Deep sources such as orbitofrontal cortex, insula, and posterior cingulate may produce little or misleading scalp change, while rapid propagation may make a remote symptomatogenic zone look like the onset itself.

Fifth, focal and generalized epilepsies can partially imitate each other semeiologically. Tufenkjian & Lüders note that focal epilepsy may trigger seizures of apparently generalized semiology, whereas generalized epilepsies can show focal-looking features such as unilateral clonic movement, version, or asymmetric tonic posturing. Semiology alone therefore cannot always separate focal from generalized epilepsy.

Sixth, the evidence base for many subregions remains limited. The SMA meta-analysis explicitly grades the certainty of the anatomo-clinical association as low to very low overall because the literature is dominated by small series and case reports despite high-quality invasive localization in many cases. The precuneus and posterior cingulate literatures remain especially sparse, meaning that highly specific claims should be avoided even when the qualitative patterns are attractive.

Seventh, surgical series are inherently selected populations. Many papers are based on presurgical cohorts or postoperative seizure-free populations. These populations enrich for focal, often unilateral, often lesional or at least surgically tractable epilepsies. Their semiologic distributions may not generalize directly to all-comers in outpatient practice.

Eighth, age modifies semiology. The pediatric hand posture paper notes that the young brain tends to spread activity rapidly and may express less differentiated distal postures than older patients. Thus, adult semiologic rules cannot always be transplanted unchanged into early childhood epilepsy.

Ninth, language, consciousness, and memory are difficult to assess reliably during seizures. Apparent preserved awareness may simply reflect a seizure too brief to test properly, and a patient's later recall may be incomplete. Similarly, dysphasia is easy to overcall unless structured testing during the seizure confirms impaired language rather than reduced responsiveness or motor speech block.

Finally, some of the most memorable semiologic signs have excellent lateralizing value but poor localizing value. Version, figure-of-four, last clonic jerk, Todd paresis, unilateral blinking, and many autonomic signs are best treated as side markers embedded within an already broader lobe hypothesis. Overusing them as lobar localizers is a common analytic error.

12.1 Practical safeguards against semiologic overinterpretation

- Always reconstruct the seizure as a timeline rather than as a bag of signs.
- Treat the earliest aura and first objective sign as primary evidence; later manifestations are secondary evidence.
- Insist on strict definitions for version, dystonia, automatisms, and impaired awareness.
- State explicitly when a feature likely reflects spread rather than onset.
- Use multimodal concordance—MRI, PET, ictal EEG, invasive EEG, and neuropsychology—as the final adjudicating framework.
- Document uncertainty honestly when competing semiologic interpretations remain plausible.

12.2 What semiology still does exceptionally well

Despite all of these limitations, the literature reviewed makes a compelling case that semiology remains indispensable. It is often the only tool that directly describes the patient's actual ictal physiology at the bedside. It guides where to place invasive electrodes, which alternative syndromes to consider, which hemisphere to suspect, and which MRI or PET findings deserve renewed attention. The correct conclusion is not that semiology is weak, but that it is powerful only when used in a disciplined, sequential, multimodal way.

Clinical takeaway

- Main safeguard: reconstruct the timeline, use strict definitions, and state uncertainty honestly.
- Best use: semiology is strongest for early symptomatogenic inference and selected lateralizing signs.
- Common trap: mistaking symptomatogenic cortex for the seizure-onset zone or epileptogenic zone.
- Final adjudication still belongs to multimodal concordance.

CHAPTER 13

Integrated Practical Conclusions

Across the literature, the most durable principle is that onset matters more than spectacle. The first symptom or first visible sign usually contains the highest-yield anatomical information, while the rest of the seizure explains the network into which the onset has propagated.

For frontal lobe epilepsy, interpret the first motor vector: focal clonus suggests precentral cortex; asymmetric bilateral tonic posturing suggests SMA recruitment; early true version suggests frontal eye field involvement, especially when it occurs early; hypermotor, vocal, fearful, or pouting patterns suggest mesiofrontal/anterior cingulate-orbitofrontal participation.

For temporal lobe epilepsy, let the aura lead the analysis: epigastric rising, déjà vu, and experiential aura point mesial; elementary auditory aura points lateral temporal/Heschl; mixed visual or vertiginous onset raises temporal-plus or temporo-occipital involvement; early language disturbance suggests dominant lateral temporal recruitment.

For parietal and insular epilepsies, take subjective onset symptoms seriously: focal contralateral paresthesia, painful or thermal aura, body schema distortion, kinetopsia, vestibular disturbance, laryngeal constriction, and broad visceral-somatosensory mixtures all deserve explicit anatomo-clinical weighting.

For occipital epilepsy, a carefully characterized visual aura often does more than any later sign. For cingulate and posterior cingulate epilepsies, propagation pattern often explains why the seizure mimics other lobes.

Clinical takeaway

- Sequence-first interpretation should remain the default habit across all lobes and networks.
- Earliest symptoms and signs outrank later propagated features.
- Lateralizing signs and localizing signs serve different roles and should not be conflated.
- When semiology, imaging, and EEG conflict, multimodal concordance should arbitrate the final hypothesis.

For lateralization, early true version, unilateral dystonia, unilateral tonic or clonic onset, figure-of-four, last clonic jerk, Todd paresis, language dominance signs, and selected autonomic/non-dominant temporal markers remain the highest-yield bedside tools.

The best clinical habit, therefore, is not to ask 'what lobe does this seizure look like?' but 'what happened first, what happened next, and which parts of the sequence likely reflect onset versus spread?' That shift in method is the core practical message of the uploaded papers.

APPENDIX A

Practical Semiologic Analysis Template

Appendix roadmap: Appendix A, Appendix H, and Appendix F function as practical workflow tools; Appendices B, G, and I are quick-reference tools for conference use; Appendices C and J summarize the supporting evidence; Appendices E and K focus on recurrent pitfalls and shared terminology.

The following template can be copied into presurgical case review notes, multidisciplinary conference worksheets, or seizure-by-seizure video-EEG reports.

A. Baseline context

- Age at onset, seizure frequency, wake/sleep distribution, habitual triggers, family video availability.
- Level of baseline language dominance certainty and handedness.
- Known lesion, PET asymmetry, scalp EEG hypothesis, prior surgical history.

B. Earliest subjective symptom

- Exact patient wording.
- Body location, hemifield, modality (visual, auditory, somatic, vestibular, experiential, autonomic, visceral).
- Was awareness preserved during the aura? Was recall reliable afterward?

C. Earliest objective sign

- Eye/head deviation, blinking, face involvement, unilateral limb sign, tonic/dystonic posture, speech impairment, behavioral arrest.
- Latency from electroclinical onset to the first objective sign.

D. Early evolving features

- Figure 20. Automatisms: oral, manual, gestural, vocal.
- Motor sequence: clonic → tonic, tonic → version, sensory → tonic, etc.
- Awareness testing results during the seizure.

E. Late ictal features

- Secondary generalization, figure-of-four, ictal-end head position, last clonic jerk.
- Features likely attributable to spread rather than onset.

F. Postictal features

- Todd paresis, aphasia, confusion, postictal nose wipe, and memory for onset.
- Duration of postictal deficits.

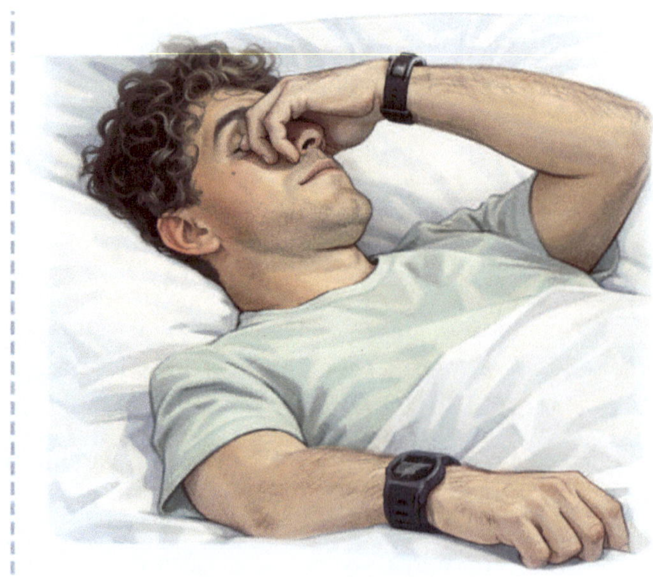

Figure 21. Patient with left temporal lobe epilepsy. Nose wiping within the first 10 seconds of the postictal period.

G. Final semiologic synthesis

- Most likely symptomatogenic zone.
- Most likely side of onset.
- Leading alternative explanation and why it remains plausible.
- Implication for invasive electrode placement.

APPENDIX B

Sublobar Semiology Matrices

Subregion	Most helpful onset semiology	Lateralization	Key pitfall
Primary motor cortex	Contralateral focal clonus/myoclonus/tonus; Jacksonian march	Contralateral	Late tonic or version may reflect spread
SMA	Asymmetric bilateral tonic posture; fencing; early tonic pattern	Extended arm contralateral	Can be recruited secondarily from parietal/occipital onset
Pre-SMA	Speech inhibition, automatisms, versive elements reported but less secure	Variable; rely on associated motor signs	Evidence sparse
Frontal eye field / DLPFC	Early true version	Contralateral	Needs strict distinction from nonversive turning
Orbitofronta l	Impaired awareness, automatisms, olfactory aura, autonomic features	Limited	May mimic parasomnia/PNES
Anterior cingulate / mesiofrontal	Fear, vocalization, screaming, hypermotor, ictal pout	From associated unilateral motor signs	May mimic temporal fear or generic frontal hypermotor epilepsy
Frontal operculum / Broca	Face clonus, laryngeal symptoms, salivation, dysphasia	Dominant hemisphere if aphasic	Overlap with insula/perisylvian network
Subregion	Most helpful onset semiology	Lateralization	Key pitfall
Mesial temporal	Epigastric rising, déjà vu, fear, behavioral arrest, oral/manual automatisms	Dystonia contralateral; preserved awareness and ictal speech favor non-dominant	Late version and late tonic signs reflect spread
Amygdala	Early apnoea, tachycardia, affective-autonomic onset	From accompanying unilateral signs	Can mimic insular autonomic onset
Lateral temporal / Heschl	Elementary auditory aura; early ictal dysphasia if dominant	Unilateral auditory aura contralateral	Can be mislabeled mesial if later automatisms dominate
Temporal pole	Temporal aura with unusually early LOC or hypermotor evolution	Uses general temporal lateralizers	Can mimic frontal epilepsy
Temporal-plus	Visual hallucinations, vertigo, hybrid posterior sensory onset followed by temporal automotor pattern	Depends on individual sign	Under-recognized if only middle phase is reviewed
Subregion	Most helpful onset semiology	Lateralization	Key pitfall

Subregion	Most helpful onset semiology	Lateralization	Key pitfall
Postcentral gyrus	Contralateral tingling/numbness; sensory march	Contralateral	Late clonus may shift attention to motor cortex
S2 / parietal operculum	Broad unpleasant somatosensory aura, heat, pain, inability to move contralateral limb	Often contralateral but less tidy	Overlap with posterior insula
SPL / intraparietal sulcus	Kinetopsia, body schema change, spatial distortion	Often difficult	Late tonic/eye deviation may falsely suggest frontal onset
Precuneus	Vestibular onset, macropsia/micropsia, altered visual/body perception	Often difficult	Rapid frontal spread can mislead
Inferior parietal / TPJ	Autoscopy, vestibular-self disturbance, reading/writing impairment	Dominant hemisphere if language involved	Overlap with temporal experiential phenomena
Primary visual cortex	Elementary visual aura, brief flashing lights	Contralateral hemifield	May be mistaken for migraine
Visual association occipital	Complex visual hallucinations, size distortion, motion illusion	Variable unless hemifield	Can be mislabeled temporal
Parieto-occipital junction	Blinking, nystagmus, eye deviation with posterior onset	Blinking ipsilateral; nystagmus fast phase contralateral	May be misread as frontal eye field onset
Subregion	Most helpful onset semiology	Lateralization	Key pitfall
Anterior cingulate	Fear, screaming, vocalization, autonomic activation, hypermotor	From associated unilateral motor signs	Can mimic temporal fear or generic frontal hypermotor
dPCC	Dizziness/vertigo, subtle posterior self-motion or visual blurring	Usually limited	Symptoms may look nonspecific
vPCC	Behavioral arrest + autonomic/epigastric phenomena + later automatisms	Usually limited	May mimic mesial temporal epilepsy
RSC	Visual/vestibular posterior symptoms with later integrated complex motor behavior	Usually limited	Late complex motor behavior may be misread as frontal onset

APPENDIX C

Paper-by-Paper Evidence Summaries

Chowdhury et al., 2021. Localisation in focal epilepsy: a practical guide

Role in this review: principal practical synthesis and organizing backbone.

- Explains the distinction among symptomatogenic zone, seizure onset zone, and epileptogenic zone.
- Emphasizes that semiology evolves with propagation and that scalp EEG reflects recruitment rather than necessarily the behavior of the underlying cortex.

- Provides lobe-by-lobe practical descriptions for frontal, temporal, parietal, occipital, cingulate, insular, and selected reflex/special seizures.
- Highlights robust lateralizing signs including early version, unilateral clonic/tonic/dystonic signs, figure-of-four, last clonic jerk, Todd paresis, unilateral blinking, and hemifield visual aura.
- Useful numerical anchors include abdominal aura probabilities in temporal lobe epilepsy and broad differentiating features between frontal and temporal seizures.

Tufenkjian & Lüders, 2012. Seizure semiology: its value and limitations in localizing the epileptogenic zone

Role in this review: methodological and cautionary framework.

- States criteria for an ideal localizing sign: reproducible, early in the seizure, and linked to a well-defined symptomatogenic zone.
- Provides a structured classification of aura types, motor seizures, dialeptic seizures, and special lateralizing signs.
- Strongly emphasizes inter-rater variability and the risk of overinterpreting late propagated signs.
- Highlights that semiology reflects symptomatogenic cortex and cannot always distinguish focal from generalized epilepsy.
- Contains clinically durable discussions of version, dystonia, postictal signs, unilateral blinking, and ictal nystagmus.

Buonocore et al., 2026. Ictal semiology in supplementary motor area and pre-SMA epilepsy

Role in this review: best dedicated synthesis for mesial frontal motor epilepsy.

- Systematic review/meta-analysis of 20 studies with extractable data from 37 patients.
- Asymmetric tonic posturing was the most frequent feature (47%), followed by automatisms (25%), version (23%), loss of consciousness (19%), sensory phenomena (11%), and speech inhibition (10%).
- Stresses that classic SMA signs are helpful but absent in many patients.
- Shows that evidence for separating SMA from pre-SMA remains limited and that invasive EEG is usually required.

Yan et al., 2024. Posterior cingulate epilepsy using SEEG

Role in this review: defining source for posterior cingulate subregional semiology.

- Analyzed 59 seizures in 15 patients with SEEG-defined posterior cingulate epilepsy.
- Behavioral arrest predominated across posterior cingulate subregions.
- Automatisms were especially linked to ventral PCC seizures spreading to temporal structures.
- Retrosplenial cortex was associated with complex motor behavior and strong visual/vestibular stimulation responses.
- Explains why posterior cingulate epilepsy so often mimics temporal or frontal epilepsy.

Sivaji et al., 2025. Initial, mid-ictal, and ictal-end head position in versive seizures

Role in this review: timing-based refinement of version interpretation.

- Shows that latency from seizure onset to version differs by lobe: earliest in frontal, latest in occipital seizures.
- Supports using very early version as a clue favoring frontal onset.
- Identifies late ictal-end head position opposite the initial version and ipsilateral to the epileptogenic zone in a subset of secondarily generalized seizures.
- Reinforces the need to distinguish true version from natural head turning.

Menderes et al., 2025. Hand postures in pediatric epilepsy

Role in this review: pediatric lateralizing adjunct.

- Fist posture was most often frontal; thumb-upside fist most often temporal; fanning most often generalized.
- Ipsilateral hand posture was more common in frontal seizures, contralateral in temporal seizures.
- Reminds the reader that ontogeny modifies semiologic expression in children and that pediatric spread can be rapid.

Khoja et al., 2021. Temporal lobe vs temporal-plus epilepsy

Role in this review: refinement of temporal border-zone interpretation.

- Highlights visual hallucinations and vertigo as features associated with temporal-plus epilepsy.
- Shows that some classic temporal motor features such as automatisms and late dystonic posture can still occur in temporal-plus cases but are more typical of conventional temporal lobe epilepsy when they dominate the sequence.
- Useful as a warning against collapsing posterior sensory onset into 'temporal' solely because automatisms appear later.

Precuneus systematic review

Role in this review: focused support for medial parietal onset patterns.

- Vestibular symptoms were the commonest onset symptoms.
- Visual illusions and body perception disturbances were also frequent.
- Motor phenomena tended to appear during propagation rather than at onset.
- Supports the concept that rapid frontal spread can obscure medial parietal origin.

Occipital lobe epilepsy surgical series

Role in this review: practical reminder of OLE heterogeneity and migraine mimicry.

- Visual aura was the commonest initial symptom.
- Secondary generalization was not rare.
- The study emphasizes that neuroimaging and invasive data often complement, rather than replace, careful clinical interpretation.

Localized pain in parietal lobe seizures

Role in this review: focused evidence that pain can be ictal and posterior in origin.

- Pain was rare but when present early and clearly ictal, parietal involvement was prominent.

- Lateralized pain pointed contralaterally to seizure onset.
- Clinically important for avoiding years of misdiagnosis.

Fotedar et al., 2022. A descriptive study of eye and head movements in versive seizures

Role in this review: focused refinement of versive semiology beyond simple left-right lateralization.

- Reaffirms that version is highly lateralizing when defined strictly as forced, sustained, and unnatural eye-head deviation.
- Shows that spontaneous versive eye movements are usually conjugate, contralateral, saccadic, and obliquely upward rather than purely horizontal.
- Notes that head deviation accompanies eye deviation in almost all cases and that ipsilateral facial motor activity is common, strengthening the frontal eye field-plus-nearby-face-motor interpretation.
- Useful clinically for refining bedside description of version rather than using version as a binary present-or-absent sign.

Fayerstein et al., 2020. Quantitative analysis of hyperkinetic seizures and correlation with seizure onset zone

Role in this review: structured SEEG-based evidence that hyperkinetic seizures are not anatomically synonymous with frontal onset.

- Introduces a 10-item Hyperkinetic Seizure Scale with good interrater agreement for symmetry, dystonia, emotion, vocalization, aura, delay, stereotypy, and integrated behavior.
- Cluster 1 - asymmetric or unilateral hyperkinetic movement with marked dystonia and aura - mainly correlated with parietal seizures.
- Cluster 2 - bilateral symmetric stereotyped hyperkinesia without dystonia - mapped to temporal and dorsolateral prefrontal seizures.
- Cluster 3 - emotional, vocal, integrated bilateral hyperkinesia - was most closely linked to ventromedial prefrontal seizures but also common in temporal hyperkinetic seizures.
- Clinically important because it argues against equating hyperkinetic behavior with frontal onset and encourages finer bedside subclassification.

Hirsch et al., 1998. Postictal nosewiping lateralizes and localizes to the ipsilateral temporal lobe

Role in this review: validation of a simple postictal bedside behavior with useful temporal and lateralizing value.

- Postictal nosewiping within 60 seconds was more common in unilateral temporal lobe epilepsy than in extratemporal epilepsy.
- When unilateral in temporal lobe epilepsy, the wiping hand was usually ipsilateral to seizure onset, and repetitive same-hand nosewiping within a single seizure was always ipsilateral in this cohort.
- The proposed mechanism links temporal-amygdalar autonomic activation with nasal secretions or sensation as awareness returns postictally.
- Best used as a supportive postictal temporal-side marker rather than as a stand-alone lobe localizer.

References

Buonocore S, Pommella M, Bettiol A, De Masi S, Barba C. Ictal semiology in supplementary motor area and pre-supplementary motor area epilepsy: A systematic review and meta-analysis. Epileptic Disorders. 2026;28:33–42.

Chowdhury FA, Silva R, Whatley B, Walker MC. Localisation in focal epilepsy: a practical guide. Practical Neurology. 2021;21:481–492.

Fayerstein J, McGonigal A, Pizzo F, Bonini F, Lagarde S, Braquet A, Trebuchon A, Carron R, Scavarda D, Julia S, Lambert I, Giusiano B, Bartolomei F. Quantitative analysis of hyperkinetic seizures and correlation with seizure onset zone. Epilepsia. 2020;61:1019-1026.

Fotedar N, Gajera P, Pyatka N, Nasralla S, Kubota T, Fernandez-Baca Vaca G, Shaikh AG, Luders HO. A descriptive study of eye and head movements in versive seizures. Seizure. 2022;98:44-50.

Hirsch LJ, Lain AH, Walczak TS. Postictal nosewiping lateralizes and localizes to the ipsilateral temporal lobe. Epilepsia. 1998;39(9):991-997.

Gardella E, Rubboli G, Tassinari CA. Ictal grasping: prevalence and characteristics in seizures with different semiology. Epilepsia. 2006;47(Suppl 5):59–63.

Ignatius E, Metsähonkala L, Jonsson H, et al. Ictal semiology in precuneus seizures: a systematic review. Epileptic Disorders. 2024.

Khoja A, Albaradei O, Alsulami A, et al. Seizure semiology in temporal lobe vs. temporal plus epilepsy using intracranial EEG monitoring. Neurosciences. 2021;26(3):261–269.

Lee SK, Lee SY, Kim DW, Lee DS, Chung CK. Occipital lobe epilepsy: clinical characteristics, surgical outcome, and role of diagnostic modalities. Epilepsia. 2005;46:686–695.

Menderes D, Hirfanoglu T, Serdaroglu E, Serdaroglu A, Arhan E. Evaluation of lateralization and localization value of hand postures in pediatric epilepsy. Seizure. 2025;127:71–76.

Saint-Hilaire JM, Lee MA. Localizing and lateralizing value of epileptic symptoms in temporal lobe epilepsy. Canadian Journal of Neurological Sciences. 2000;27(Suppl 1):S1–S5.

Siegel AM, Williamson PD, Roberts DW, Thadani VM, Darcey TM. Localized pain associated with seizures originating in the parietal lobe. Epilepsia. 1999;40(7).

Sivaji AR, Nazam I, Thyagaraj S, Fotedar N. Localizing and lateralizing significance of initial, mid-ictal, and ictal-end head position in versive seizures with secondary generalization. Neurology Clinical Practice. 2025;15:e200559.

Tufenkjian K, Lüders HO. Seizure semiology: its value and limitations in localizing the epileptogenic zone. Journal of Clinical Neurology. 2012;8:243–250.

Wan H, Zhao X, Fu W, et al. Anatomo-electro-clinical features of parietal lobe epilepsy: insights from scalp video-electroencephalography. CNS Neuroscience & Therapeutics. 2026.

Yan Z, Yang Y, Wang J, et al. Posterior cingulate epilepsy: seizure semiology and intracranial electrical stimulation using SEEG. Seizure. 2024;119:28–35.

APPENDIX D

Sign-Oriented Compendium

This appendix inverts the lobe-based organization of the main text. Instead of asking where seizures begin, it asks what a specific sign usually means, how much weight it deserves, and how the same sign can mislead the interpreter if timing is ignored. The goal is to support real-world video review in which the observer first notices a symptom and then needs to work backward toward plausible anatomy.

Somatosensory aura

A clearly focal somatosensory aura remains one of the highest-yield localizing symptoms in focal epilepsy when it is early, reproducible, and anatomically described with precision. Distal unilateral tingling or numbness points first toward contralateral primary sensory cortex. When the sensation marches across adjacent body parts, the argument for postcentral onset becomes even stronger. By contrast, bilateral, diffuse, or whole-body sensations are much less useful and may arise from supplementary sensorimotor regions, secondary sensory cortex, posterior insula, or even from nonspecific spread. The critical practical distinction is therefore not simply whether a seizure has a somatosensory aura, but whether the aura is topographically disciplined or anatomically vague.

The main pitfall is that motor cortex stimulation at low intensity can be perceived subjectively as somatic sensation, and posterior insula/S2 can produce broad, painful, or thermal sensations that look superficially similar to postcentral onset. A small, distal, contralateral, marching aura deserves higher localizing weight than a large or bilateral discomfort. When the same seizure later becomes tonic, clonic, or automotor, that late evolution should be treated as spread unless the initial sensory symptom was absent or unreliable.

Pain and thermal aura

Pain is unusual but deeply localizing when it is genuinely ictal and begins early. The uploaded parietal pain paper reminds us that unilateral peripheral pain, cephalic pain, and even abdominal pain can arise from parietal-onset seizures. The practical guide also places painful and thermal sensations in secondary sensory cortex and posterior insula. Therefore, early pain should immediately prompt a posterior network hypothesis rather than a default temporal interpretation. Burning, electric, hot, or shock-like sensations that involve broad or unusual territories especially support posterior insular or S2-opercular participation.

The main pitfall is to dismiss painful seizures as psychogenic, musculoskeletal, or migrainous. The second pitfall is to assume that abdominal pain must be temporal. When abdominal pain appears as an early, stereotyped ictal manifestation, posterior parietal-insular pathways should remain in consideration.

Visual aura

Visual aura is only as useful as its description. Elementary positive visual phenomena—flashing lights, bright spots, simple shapes, colored lights, often brief and stereotyped—point toward primary visual cortex. Complex visual phenomena such as formed hallucinations, motion illusions, macropsia, micropsia, and autoscopy imply higher-order visual association or temporo-parieto-occipital network involvement. Hemifield visual symptoms are especially valuable because they lateralize contralaterally. Diffuse or binocular visual change is still consistent with occipital epilepsy but carries less side certainty.

The major pitfall is migraine. Duration, stereotypy, and subsequent epileptic evolution are the practical discriminators. Another pitfall is to interpret all complex visual phenomena as temporal simply because they are 'elaborate'; the uploaded papers repeatedly show that occipital and parietal networks can generate very sophisticated visual disturbances.

Auditory aura

Simple auditory aura—buzzing, humming, ringing, or noise—remains a high-yield sign for lateral temporal neocortex, particularly Heschl gyrus. When unilateral, it supports a contralateral focus. Complex auditory experiences such as voices, music, or distortion suggest auditory association cortex and may broaden the differential toward lateral temporal, temporoparietal, or insular networks. In practical video-EEG interpretation, the auditory aura is often overlooked because it is brief and subjective; direct post-seizure questioning is therefore essential.

The main pitfall is poor lateralization by patient report. Many patients experience the sound as 'in both ears' or cannot reliably assign side. Auditory aura should also be distinguished from non-epileptic tinnitus and from the rising inner-noise sensation some patients describe with anxiety or presyncope.

Olfactory and gustatory aura

Olfactory and gustatory auras are classically associated with mesial temporal and insular networks, with orbitofrontal cortex also contributing to olfactory semiology. In the uploaded papers they are useful because they are relatively specific for focal epilepsy and because they shift the differential away from frontal hypermotor or primary sensory-motor syndromes. Gustatory symptoms especially support insular participation, whereas olfactory aura may fit mesial temporal, insular, or orbitofrontal onset depending on the total sequence.

The pitfall is low side value. These auras help localization by network class more than by hemisphere. If later temporal automatisms appear, mesial temporal onset becomes more plausible; if the aura is accompanied by laryngeal constriction, salivation, or broad somatic discomfort, insular involvement rises.

Abdominal aura

No aura in the uploaded set is more practically important than the abdominal or epigastric rising sensation. It is strongly associated with temporal lobe epilepsy, especially mesial temporal onset, and its evolution into an automotor seizure markedly strengthens that interpretation. Yet the same literature warns against dogmatism: abdominal auras can also arise from insular, frontal, and posterior cingulate/peri-limbic networks. The practical solution is sequence-based weighting. A clean epigastric rising sensation followed by behavioral arrest and oral-manual automatisms still strongly supports mesial temporal onset. An epigastric or visceral discomfort accompanied at once by laryngeal, salivatory, or broad somatic-autonomic features should raise insular or ventral posterior cingulate possibilities.

The pitfall is assuming that one symptom overrides the rest of the sequence. In presurgical patients, abdominal aura should trigger careful review of all early associated features rather than automatic mesial temporal labeling.

Autonomic aura and autonomic seizures

Autonomic symptoms are among the least appreciated and most network-rich semiologies in focal epilepsy. Tachycardia, piloerection, nausea, sweating, goose bumps, pallor, vomiting, or an urge to urinate may all be epileptic. In the uploaded papers, anterior insula, amygdala, cingulate, and non-dominant temporal structures all participate in autonomic semiology. The practical question is therefore not whether autonomic symptoms are localizing on their own, but what they accompany. Tachycardia plus fear plus hypermotor behavior supports anterior cingulate/mesiofrontal recruitment. Tachycardia or apnoea in a classic experiential-visceral temporal sequence suggests amygdalar participation. Nausea plus laryngeal constriction and hypersalivation points toward anterior insula. Peri-ictal drinking, spitting, vomiting, or urge to urinate may support non-dominant temporal involvement.

The main pitfall is overuse of autonomic symptoms as side markers. Most autonomic signs are weak for lateralization. They should guide network hypothesis rather than replace more robust motor or language asymmetries.

Psychic and experiential aura

Experiential phenomena such as déjà vu, jamais vu, fear, depersonalization, altered familiarity, and autoscopic experience remain strongly clinically informative but not always anatomically pure. Mesial temporal structures classically produce these auras, but posterior cingulate, temporoparietal, and occipito-parietal association cortex can generate overlapping symptoms. The most useful interpretive habit is to distinguish pure familiarity/emotional experience from body-self or visual-spatial distortion. Pure déjà vu plus epigastric rising plus later automatisms still strongly supports mesial temporal epilepsy. Déjà vu with dizziness, visual haze, or posterior perceptual complaints should raise posterior cingulate or precuneus possibilities.

The pitfall is to call every unusual conscious experience 'temporal'. The uploaded posterior cingulate study is particularly helpful as a warning against that error.

Dialeptic onset

Behavioral arrest and loss of responsiveness can be profoundly misleading if treated as a localizer without context. Temporal lobe epilepsy often produces dialeptic seizures, but dialeptic onset can also result from posterior cingulate spread, frontal network recruitment, and other distributed patterns. The key is to ask what happened just before the arrest and what happened immediately after it. In temporal lobe epilepsy, dialepsis is often preceded by aura and followed by automatisms with more prolonged postictal confusion. In posterior cingulate epilepsy, the dialeptic component may be an early manifestation of deep network engagement before temporal-like spread becomes apparent.

The pitfall is to treat behavioral arrest as a generic sign of temporal lobe onset. Its anatomical meaning depends entirely on sequence.

Automotor behavior

Oral and manual automatisms are strongly associated with temporal lobe epilepsy, but they are not temporal-exclusive. Frontal, posterior cingulate, and temporal-plus epilepsies may all evolve into automotor behavior after spread to temporal circuits. The most reliable temporal use of automatisms is therefore contextual: when they follow mesial temporal aura and behavioral arrest, they strongly support temporal onset. When they appear after posterior sensory or vestibular symptoms, they may represent propagation.

The pitfall is to define the seizure by its middle phase instead of by its onset. Invasive EEG failures often begin with this bedside analytic error.

Hypermotor behavior

Hypermotor seizures often suggest frontal or anterior cingulate networks, especially when abrupt, sleep-related, and accompanied by fear, vocalization, or semipurposeful proximal movements. Yet the uploaded literature also reminds the reader that temporal pole, temporal-plus, insular, and posterior cingulate seizures can become hypermotor after spread. The most localizing use of hypermotor behavior is therefore when it is early, abrupt, and not preceded by a well-formed posterior or visceral aura.

The pitfall is to anchor too early on a frontal label. Hypermotor behavior is highly visible but not always where the seizure begins.

Tonic posturing

Tonic posturing has excellent lateralizing value when clearly unilateral and strong pattern value when asymmetric and bilateral, but only moderate onset specificity. Asymmetric bilateral tonic posturing is the flagship sign of SMA epilepsy, especially when abrupt and early. However, the practical guide repeatedly warns that parietal and occipital seizures may produce tonic posturing after spread to the SMA. Therefore, tonic posturing localizes best when it is the first objective sign and when the pre-ictal history lacks a more anatomically specific sensory or experiential onset.

The pitfall is overcalling mesial frontal onset in any seizure with tonic posturing.

Clonic activity

Contralateral focal clonic activity remains among the cleanest bedside localizers when it appears at onset. It usually points toward primary motor cortex or nearby perirolandic spread. Later clonic activity during a convulsive seizure remains useful for lateralization, especially when the last clonic jerk is asymmetric, but loses onset-localizing purity.

The pitfall is timing blindness. Early focal clonus and late clonic participation mean different things.

Version and ocular signs

True version is among the most validated lateralizing signs in epilepsy, but only under strict definition. Early forced version is contralateral and, when very early, raises frontal onset probability. Posterior seizures may also produce ocular signs, however, especially when occipital or parieto-occipital networks are involved. Nystagmus, unilateral blinking, and eye deviation therefore require careful separation from frontal eye field version. Unilateral blinking tends to lateralize ipsilaterally; the fast phase of epileptic nystagmus usually points contralaterally.

The pitfall is to use the word 'version' loosely. Precision of terminology matters more here than in almost any other semiologic domain.

Language impairment

Aphasic disturbance during seizures can be highly useful for hemispheric dominance but less useful for lobe localization. Dominant temporal, temporoparietal, and inferior frontal networks can all produce ictal or postictal dysphasia. Speech arrest, by contrast, may arise from frontal inhibitory mechanisms and is less lateralizing. The practical bedside solution is structured testing during the seizure whenever feasible: name, repeat, read, follow verbal and non-verbal commands, and assess awareness separately from language.

The pitfall is to infer localization from reduced speech output alone.

Postictal signs

Postictal signs are often under-weighted in modern semiology even though they retain high lateralizing value. Todd paresis points contralaterally. Postictal aphasia points to the dominant hemisphere. Postictal confusion is more prominent in temporal than in frontal seizures on average. In selected temporal lobe epilepsy series, postictal nose wipe and related grooming behaviors may also carry side value, though these were not central in the uploaded broad practical guide.

The pitfall is forgetting that postictal signs lateralize side more than lobe. They should close the semiologic loop rather than define the onset region alone.

APPENDIX E

Common Mislocalization Scenarios and How to Avoid Them

1. Parietal sensory onset mislabeled as SMA epilepsy

A seizure begins with a brief contralateral tingling of the hand and then rapidly becomes asymmetric bilateral tonic. If the sensory onset is ignored, the seizure looks mesial frontal. The correction is to privilege the earliest topographic symptom and interpret the tonic phase as spread to SMA.

2. Temporal-plus epilepsy mislabeled as mesial temporal epilepsy

Visual hallucination or vertigo at onset is followed by behavioral arrest and oral-manual automatisms. The middle phase looks temporal, but the posterior sensory onset suggests a temporal-plus or temporo-occipital network.

3. Posterior cingulate epilepsy mislabeled as temporal lobe epilepsy

The seizure begins with vague dizziness, déjà vu, or epigastric discomfort and then becomes automotor. Without attention to the posterior clue and the possibility of rapid temporal recruitment, the event is assigned to mesial temporal structures too confidently.

4. Insular onset mislabeled as mesial temporal due to abdominal aura

A visceral rising sensation is accompanied by throat tightness, hypersalivation, or broad somatic discomfort. These additional features should prevent automatic mesial temporal labeling.

5. Occipital epilepsy mislabeled as migraine

The patient reports recurrent brief flashing colored lights followed by eye deviation and later altered awareness. The brevity, stereotypy, and ictal evolution support epilepsy over migraine aura.

6. Frontal hypermotor seizure mislabeled as psychogenic event

The seizure is bizarre, abrupt, nocturnal, and poorly localizing on scalp EEG. Orbitofrontal or mesiofrontal origin should remain in the differential when the event is stereotyped and brief.

7. Version overused as a frontal localizer

A seizure with late version after sensory or experiential onset should not be localized to the frontal eye field. Version often marks spread, not origin.

8. Late automotor behavior overused as a temporal localizer

Automatisms can arise after spread from posterior cingulate, insular, parietal, or temporal-plus networks. Their interpretive weight depends on what preceded them.

9. Emotional aura overused as a mesial temporal sign

Fear can arise from mesial temporal structures but also from anterior cingulate and mesiofrontal networks. Motor-autonomic context matters.

10. Whole-body sensation treated as localizing

Poorly localized all-body sensory symptoms have little localizing value. They should not be weighted like a focal sensory march.

11. Pediatric semiology interpreted by adult rules alone

Rapid spread and developmental factors may blunt the specificity of distal or complex postures in children. Pediatric signs are useful but require age-aware caution.

12. Postictal aphasia mistaken for ictal speech arrest

Dominant hemisphere postictal aphasia has different lateralizing implications from ictal speech arrest. Timing relative to seizure termination is essential.

APPENDIX F

Relative Confidence Framework for Semiology-Based Inference

The following matrix is intended for conference discussion rather than for rigid scoring. It summarizes how much confidence semiology alone usually deserves before integration with MRI, PET, scalp EEG, and invasive EEG.

Inference type	When confidence is highest	When confidence should drop
Lobe localization	Clear early aura or elementary sign with strong anatomo-clinical correlation	Late dominant sign only, rapid spread, poor patient recall, conflicting early symptoms
Sublobar localization	Pathognomonic-type onset such as Jacksonian march, elementary visual aura, simple auditory aura, focal sensory march	Deep/mesial regions, multimodal symptoms, very brief onset, heavily propagated seizures
Hemispheric lateralizatio n	Concordant motor asymmetries (version + dystonia + figure-of-four, etc.)	Only autonomic or affective signs, or conflicting lateralizers
Language dominance inference	Structured ictal/postictal testing shows aphasia or preserved awareness with automatisms	Speech arrest without testing, impaired responsiveness alone
Network-	Posterior sensory symptom followed by temporal/frontal	Generic dialeptic or motor semiology

Inference type	When confidence is highest	When confidence should drop
level suspicion	spread; mixed visceral-somatosensory onset	without clear onset phenomenology

Suggested wording in reports: low confidence, moderate confidence, or high confidence. Reserve high confidence for cases with an anatomically specific early sign and at least one concordant non-semiologic modality.

APPENDIX G

Quick-Reference Sublobar Interpretation Cards

Interpretive pearl for all cards: document whether the pattern occurred at onset, after a specific aura, or only after the seizure had already generalized within a larger network. That temporal distinction often changes the final localization more than the sign itself.

The cards below are designed for rapid conference use. Each card condenses the most actionable anatomo-clinical message for a single subregion. The wording intentionally favors interpretive discipline over memorization of exotic signs.

Primary motor cortex

- Think here when the seizure begins with contralateral focal clonic activity or a slow Jacksonian march.
- A later tonic phase does not cancel the earlier motor-strip localization.
- Best side rule: the early clonic activity is contralateral to onset.

SMA-proper

- Think here when the first visible sign is abrupt asymmetric bilateral tonic posturing, especially fencing.
- If sensory or visual aura clearly precedes the tonic phase, consider propagated SMA recruitment rather than primary SMA onset.
- Best side rule: the extended arm usually points contralaterally.

Pre-SMA

- Think here when speech inhibition, complex motor sequencing, or frontal automatisms occur near onset without a cleaner posterior aura.
- Evidence is thinner than for SMA-proper, so confidence should remain moderate unless invasive data are concordant.
- Best side rule: derive from accompanying motor asymmetry rather than from speech block alone.

Frontal eye field

- Think here when true forced version appears very early.
- Very late version is more likely spread than onset.
- Best side rule: initial version is contralateral.

Orbitofrontal cortex

- Think here in brief sleep-related seizures with impaired awareness, automatisms, autonomic flavor, or occasional olfactory aura.
- Do not be reassured by nonlocalizing scalp EEG in a deep frontal syndrome.
- Best side rule: usually from accompanying unilateral motor signs, not from the aura alone.

Anterior cingulate

- Think here when fear, scream, vocalization, autonomic activation, and hypermotor behavior come together early.
- An early ictal pout strongly supports this network.
- Best side rule: use the unilateral motor accompaniments, not the affect alone.

Frontal operculum

- Think here when face clonus, laryngeal symptoms, salivation, and articulation difficulty cluster together.
- Figure 21. Differentiate carefully from anterior insula.
- Best side rule: language impairment supports the dominant side.

Mesial temporal lobe

- Think here when epigastric rising, déjà vu, fear, and later oral-manual automatisms define the sequence.
- The aura often tells more than the later motor phase.
- Best side rule: unilateral dystonia is contralateral; preserved awareness during automatisms favors the non-dominant side.

Figure 22. Ictal dystonia of the right hand in a patient with left temporal lobe sclerosis.

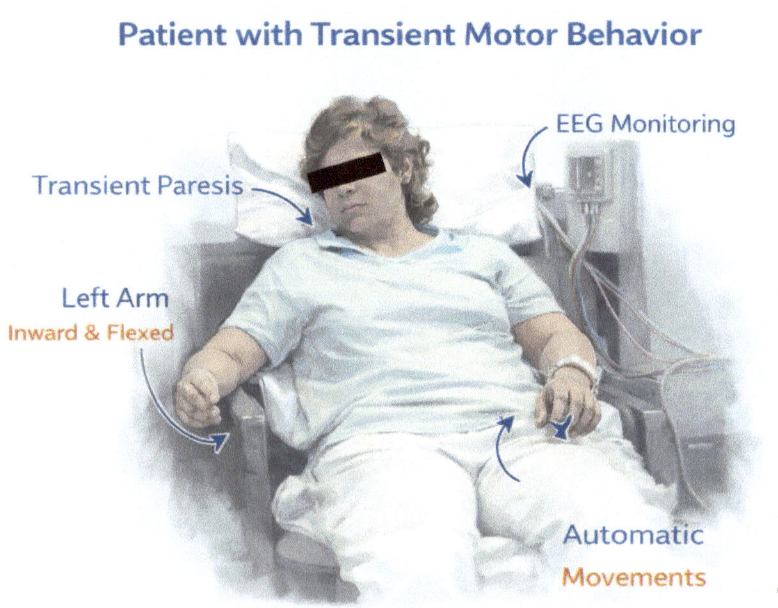

Amygdala-dominant mesial temporal pattern

- Think here when a temporal experiential aura is accompanied very early by apnoea or tachycardia.
- Autonomic richness does not automatically imply insula.
- Best side rule: side usually comes from accompanying temporal lateralizers.

Lateral temporal / Heschl gyrus

- Think here when the seizure begins with simple auditory aura or early dominant-language impairment.
- Later automatisms do not erase the lateral temporal onset clue.
- Best side rule: unilateral auditory aura is contralateral.

Temporal pole

- Think here when a temporal seizure loses awareness unusually early or becomes hypermotor early.
- This is a frequent bridge between temporal and frontal-looking semiology.
- Best side rule: same as other temporal seizures.

Temporal-plus network

- Think here when posterior sensory symptoms such as visual hallucination or vertigo lead into a temporal automotor phase.
- This diagnosis matters especially when standard temporal surgery data do not fit.
- Best side rule: follow the individual sign; the syndrome itself is not strongly lateralizing.

Anterior insula

- Think here when abdominal discomfort, laryngeal constriction, nausea, salivation, and broad body-internal sensation appear together.
- This is the seizure that most often pretends to be mesial temporal from a distance.
- Best side rule: weak from aura alone; use associated motor or sensory asymmetry.

Posterior insula

- Think here when burning, electric, painful, or unusually broad somatosensory aura appears early.
- Perioral or bilateral spread strengthens the insular hypothesis.
- Best side rule: lower confidence than in a tidy postcentral sensory march.

Postcentral gyrus

- Think here when the aura is contralateral, focal, somatotopic, and possibly marching.
- A late motor phase usually means spread forward.
- Best side rule: contralateral.

S2 / parietal operculum

- Think here when sensory aura is broad, unpleasant, painful, or includes a feeling of inability to move the contralateral limb.
- Overlap with posterior insula is expected.
- Best side rule: often contralateral but less orderly than postcentral.

Superior parietal lobule

- Think here when altered body perception or movement illusion (kinetopsia) is prominent.
- Later tonic or eye-deviation features often reflect frontal spread.
- Best side rule: often infer from associated unilateral signs rather than from the illusion itself.

Precuneus

- Think here when vestibular onset or altered visual/body scale is followed later by frontal-looking motor activity.
- The key error is to localize the seizure from the late motor phase instead of the early perceptual phase.
- Best side rule: often limited unless later unilateral signs appear.

Inferior parietal / TPJ

- Think here when autoscopy, vestibular-self disturbance, or reading/writing problems dominate onset.
- Temporal spread can make these seizures look experiential or automotor.
- Best side rule: dominant-side language signs can be especially helpful.

Primary visual cortex

- Think here when visual aura is elementary, brief, and stereotyped.
- Ask explicitly about hemifield, color, brightness, and duration.
- Best side rule: hemifield aura is contralateral.

Visual association cortex

- Think here when the visual experience is complex: formed hallucinations, motion, size change, visual scene distortion.
- These seizures can look temporal later because spread is common.
- Best side rule: lower than for elementary hemifield aura unless clearly lateralized.

Parieto-occipital junction

- Think here when blinking, nystagmus, or eye deviation accompanies a clearly posterior sensory onset.
- Differentiate ocular spread from primary frontal eye field version.
- Best side rule: blinking ipsilateral; nystagmus fast phase contralateral.

dPCC

- Think here when subtle dizziness, vertigo, or posterior self-motion symptoms precede a poorly localizing focal seizure.
- This is a deep, easily overlooked hypothesis zone.
- Best side rule: usually weak without accompanying unilateral signs.

vPCC

- Think here when behavioral arrest and autonomic/epigastric symptoms evolve almost immediately into a temporal-like automotor seizure.
- This is one of the most important temporal mimics in the uploaded set.

- Best side rule: derive from later motor asymmetry rather than the syndrome itself.

RSC

- Think here when visual/vestibular posterior symptoms are followed by integrated complex motor behavior and longer impairment of consciousness.
- Late complex motor behavior does not necessarily mean frontal onset.
- Best side rule: usually limited from syndrome alone.

APPENDIX H

High-Yield Questions to Ask During Video Review

- Was there a reportable aura before any movement occurred, and was it sensory, visual, auditory, vestibular, visceral, autonomic, or experiential?
- If the first visible sign was head turning, was it truly forced and unnatural, or could it have been a natural head movement?
- Did any unilateral limb posture appear before generalization, and which arm was extended or held in dystonia?
- Was there a focal clonic onset that later became tonic or bilateral?
- Was awareness genuinely preserved, or was the patient simply too briefly tested?
- Did language fail because of aphasia, because of speech arrest, or because of reduced responsiveness?
- Did a late temporal automotor phase obscure an earlier posterior symptom?
- Was a posterior cingulate or precuneus clue present but too subtle to dominate the bedside impression?
- If the patient described dizziness, what kind of dizziness was it: spinning, tilting, falling, detachment, or visual disorientation?
- If the patient described visual symptoms, were they positive or negative, elementary or complex, hemifield or diffuse?
- Did the seizure end with a last clonic jerk on one side, postictal weakness, or postictal aphasia?
- Was the same sequence reproducible across several habitual seizures, or are we over-interpreting a single atypical event?

This appendix deliberately converts the review into operational questions. In practice, better questions produce better semiology, and better semiology produces better invasive planning.

APPENDIX I

Comprehensive Sign Matrix for Conference Use

This matrix is intentionally redundant with the main review. Its purpose is speed during multidisciplinary discussion. Each row answers four questions: where the sign points, whether it helps with side, what usually confounds it, and how aggressively it should be weighted when the sign is early versus late.

Sign	Main localizing implication	Main side implication	Main confounder or caution

Sign	Main localizing implication	Main side implication	Main confounder or caution
Epigastric rising	Mesial temporal > ventral PCC / insula / frontal-limbic network	Usually little direct side value	Late visceral spread; nonspecific nausea
Déjà vu / jamais vu	Mesial temporal but also posterior cingulate / TPJ	Low side value	Treat with caution if posterior symptoms coexist
Simple auditory aura	Lateral temporal / Heschl gyrus	Contralateral if truly unilateral	Patient often cannot lateralize the sound
Complex auditory aura	Lateral temporal association / temporoparietal / insular	Usually low	May be misread as psychiatric or subjective noise
Elementary visual aura	Primary visual cortex	Contralateral if hemifield	Migraine aura if duration is ignored
Complex visual hallucination	Visual association cortex / TPO network	Variable	Can be mislabeled temporal
Macropsia / micropsia	Precuneus or visual association cortex	Usually low	May be called dissociative if poorly elicited
Kinetopsia	SPL / intraparietal sulcus	Usually low	Later spread can create frontal-looking seizures
Vertigo / vestibular aura	Parietal, TPJ, precuneus, dPCC/RSC, lateral temporal	Usually limited	Needs detailed phenomenology; dizziness is not one sign
Laryngeal constriction	Anterior insula / frontal operculum	Low	May be mistaken for panic or reflux
Hypersalivation	Anterior insula / frontal operculum / non-dominant temporal spread	Usually low	Often appears after spread
Painful aura	Posterior insula / S2 / parietal network	Contralateral if clearly unilateral	Frequently overlooked as epileptic
Somatosensory march	Primary sensory cortex	Contralateral	Loss of value if the initial march is uncertain
Behavioral arrest	Temporal, posterior cingulate, propagated focal seizure	Minimal by itself	Needs onset context
Oral automatisms	Temporal spread or onset	Limited; preserved awareness favors non-dominant	Can appear after posterior spread
Manual automatisms	Temporal, ventral PCC spread, frontal/complex spread	Limited	Do not let middle phase override onset aura
Hypermotor behavior	Frontal / anterior cingulate / orbitofrontal / temporal pole / spread	Low by itself	Highly visible but often late
Asymmetric bilateral tonic posturing	SMA recruitment	Extended arm contralateral	Onset may still be parietal or occipital with spread
Unilateral tonic posturing	Motor or premotor network	Contralateral	Time it carefully relative to onset
Unilateral dystonia	Often temporal lobe epilepsy	Contralateral	Requires adequate duration

Sign	Main localizing implication	Main side implication	Main confounder or caution
			and clarity
Focal clonic onset	Primary motor or perirolandic onset	Contralateral	Late clonus may simply reflect spread
True version	Frontal eye field recruitment	Contralateral	Localizing value depends on latency
Version within ~15 s	Frontal onset favored	Contralateral	Only if truly versive and correctly timed
Late version	Spread to frontal eye field	Still contralateral	Poor lobe localization
Ictal-end head position opposite initial version	Seen in some secondarily generalized seizures	Ipsilateral to onset	Only useful in the specific convulsive context
Figure-of-four	Motor spread near generalization	Extended arm contralateral	Lobe value limited
Last clonic jerk	End of focal-to-bilateral tonic-clonic seizure	Ipsilateral	Not helpful for lobe
Todd paresis	Postictal marker	Contralateral	Need true weakness rather than fatigue
Ictal speech	Temporal non-dominant more typical	Non-dominant hemisphere favored	Supportive, not absolute
Ictal/postictal aphasia	Dominant hemisphere recruitment	Dominant side	Poor lobe precision
Preserved awareness with automatisms	Temporal non-dominant more likely	Non-dominant side	Requires adequate ictal testing
Unilateral blinking	Usually ocular/periorbital ictal sign	Ipsilateral	Differentiate from flutter
Epileptic nystagmus	Occipital / temporo-occipital network	Fast phase contralateral	Rare and easily missed
Ictal pout	Mesiofrontal / anterior cingulate / orbitofrontal / premotor	Little direct side value	Most useful when early
Gelastic laughter	Hypothalamic hamartoma in childhood; frontal/temporal/cingulate in adults	Low	Network sign more than a side sign
Hand fist posture	Frontal (pediatric cohort)	Often ipsilateral	Adjunct only
Thumb-upside fist	Temporal (pediatric cohort)	Often contralateral	Adjunct only
Ictal grasping	Frontal hyperkinetic seizures more typical	No reliable side value	Can be occasional purposeful movement in extrafrontal seizures

Suggested use during case conference: first identify all signs present in the seizure; second circle those that occurred before the seizure was clearly generalized or broadly propagated; third give extra weight only to those early signs with high anatomo-clinical specificity.

APPENDIX J

Annotated Bibliography of the Uploaded Papers

Chowdhury et al., 2021

This is the principal organizing paper for the review. Its value lies less in novelty than in clarity: it provides a clinically accessible framework for frontal, temporal, parietal, occipital, cingulate, and insular semiology while insisting that symptoms reflect symptomatogenic cortex rather than automatically revealing the epileptogenic zone. It is particularly strong for differential practical clues such as frontal versus temporal, the meaning of early versus late signs, and a concise atlas-like figure of symptomatogenic zones.

Figure 22. Patient seizure with EEG monitoring.

Tufenkjian & Lüders, 2012

This paper is the best methodological counterweight to the practical guide. It is especially useful for explaining why semiology both matters and misleads. Its enduring contribution is to define what makes a sign clinically trustworthy: early occurrence, reproducibility, anatomical plausibility, and observer reliability. It also preserves older but still very serviceable distinctions among aura types, dialeptic seizures, simple motor signs, and complex motor patterns.

Buonocore et al., 2026

This systematic review and meta-analysis is important because it quantifies what clinicians often overlearn qualitatively about SMA epilepsy. The finding that asymmetric tonic posturing occurs in fewer than half of confirmed cases is clinically sobering. The paper is also valuable for its candor about evidentiary limits: despite invasive localization in many cases, the literature remains small and heterogeneous.

Yan et al., 2024

This is the key paper for posterior cingulate epilepsy in the uploaded set. Its strongest contribution is not merely listing symptoms but showing how subregional posterior cingulate semiology depends on propagation. The distinction among dPCC, vPCC, and RSC gives the clinician a usable language for a syndrome that otherwise tends to dissolve into 'temporal-like' or 'frontal-like' shorthand.

Sivaji et al., 2025

This paper upgrades the interpretation of version from a simple lateralizing sign to a time-dependent sign. Its practical value is high because version is common in video review yet often interpreted too coarsely. The latency-based framework is particularly useful in separating early frontal recruitment from later propagated version and in reminding the reader that not all head turning deserves the label 'versive'.

Figure 23. Leftward head deviation 5 seconds after ictal onset in a patient with right frontal lobe epilepsy.

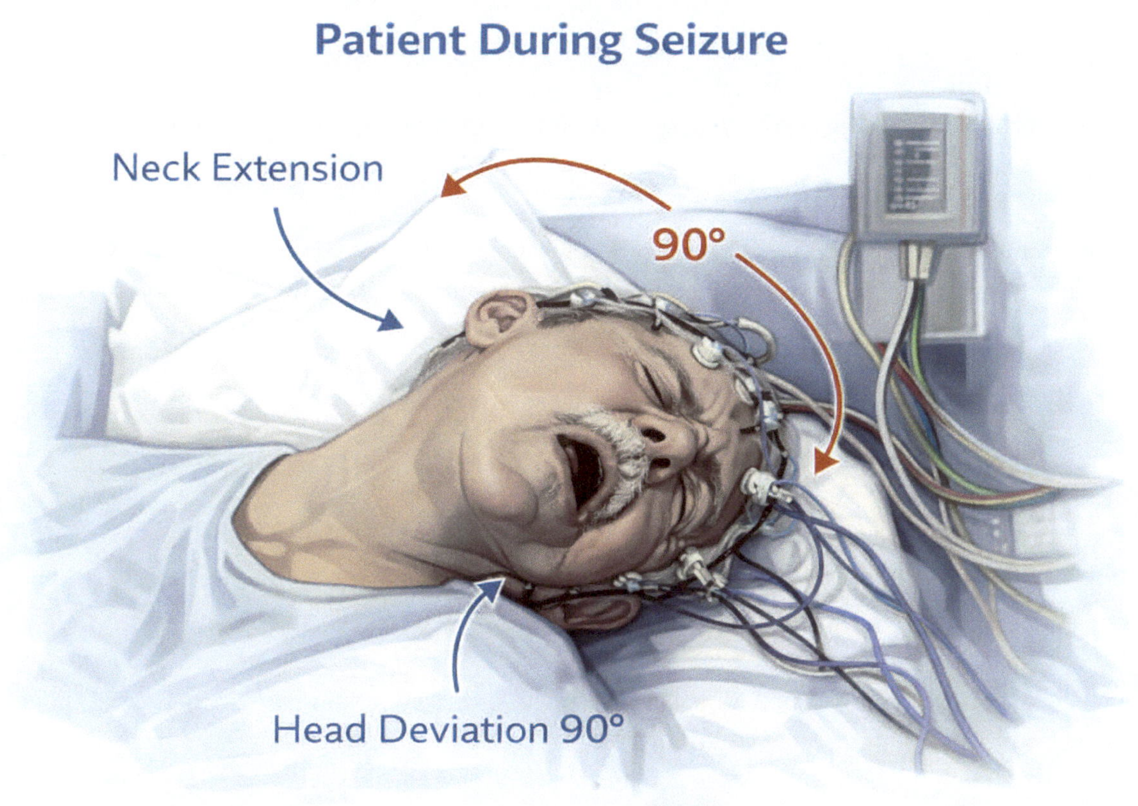

Menderes et al., 2025

This pediatric cohort is valuable because it focuses on a bedside sign that is easy to annotate from ordinary video—hand posture. Even though the study has limitations, it expands practical semiology into a domain that clinicians and families routinely observe. It also serves as a broader reminder that developmental stage alters semiologic expression.

Khoja et al., 2021

The temporal-versus-temporal-plus comparison is useful precisely because it addresses a common presurgical failure mode: assuming that the presence of automatisms settles the matter in favor of temporal onset. By highlighting visual hallucinations and vertigo in temporal-plus epilepsy, the paper helps preserve attention to posterior onset clues.

Ignatius et al., 2024

The precuneus systematic review fills a relatively underdeveloped area in focal epilepsy semiology. Its greatest value is conceptual: it teaches the clinician to expect vestibular, visual, and body-perception onset phenomena with later frontal-appearing motor evolution. That sequence is the clinical fingerprint of medial parietal epilepsy in many real cases.

Gardella et al., 2006

The ictal grasping paper adds granularity to frontal hyperkinetic semiology. Its most practical message is negative: ictal grasping is more characteristic of frontal hyperkinetic seizures than of temporal lobe epilepsy, but it is not a reliable side marker. This makes it a useful descriptive sign but not a stand-alone localizer.

Saint-Hilaire & Lee, 2000

This classic temporal lobe paper remains useful because it captures the enduring semiologic hierarchy of temporal onset: aura first, then ictal automatisms and motor signs, then postictal deficits for lateralization. It is best read as a temporal-focused complement to the broader semiology reviews.

Lee et al., 2005

The occipital surgical series is important less for narrowly localizing one occipital subregion than for demonstrating how often occipital epilepsy is clinically heterogeneous and confused with migraine. It also underscores that occipital interpretation requires integration of semiology with imaging and invasive data rather than reliance on surface appearance alone.

Siegel et al., 1999

This focused paper is clinically memorable because it validates a symptom many clinicians still under-recognize as epileptic: pain. Its main contribution is to force the epileptologist to keep painful aura within the semiologic vocabulary of focal epilepsy, especially for posterior cortical seizures.

Wan et al., 2026

The parietal scalp-video EEG paper is notable for trying to move beyond generic descriptions of parietal polymorphism toward subgrouping by anatomy. Although some of its associations should be interpreted cautiously, it is useful as a reminder that modern parietal semiology can and should be discussed in finer sublobar terms when the data allow.

Fotedar et al., 2022

This paper is valuable because it rescues version from crude yes-or-no use and restores attention to its internal motor anatomy. By showing that spontaneous versive eye movements are usually saccadic, obliquely upward, tightly coupled to head deviation, and commonly accompanied by ipsilateral facial motor activity, it gives the clinician a more realistic bedside picture of frontal eye field recruitment.

Fayerstein et al., 2020

This SEEG-based study is important because it quantifies a syndrome that clinicians often describe too loosely. Its major contribution is to show that hyperkinetic seizures sort into reproducible patterns that cut across frontal, temporal, and parietal onset zones, which makes it especially useful for differential diagnosis when a seizure looks dramatic but not anatomically pure.

Hirsch et al., 1998

This classic postictal semiology paper remains clinically useful because it validates a behavior that is easy to miss unless the reviewer watches beyond ictal offset. Its greatest practical value is not that nosewiping proves temporal onset, but that unilateral or repetitive same-hand postictal nosewiping can provide meaningful ipsilateral side information in an otherwise plausible temporal syndrome.

APPENDIX K

Glossary of Frequently Used Semiologic Terms

Automotor seizure

A seizure in which the dominant visible features are automatisms, usually oral and/or distal manual, classically associated with temporal lobe epilepsy but not specific to it.

Behavioral arrest

A cessation of ongoing behavior or responsiveness; highly common but anatomically nonspecific unless interpreted with onset context.

Chapeau de gendarme

An ictal pout with downturned mouth caused by bilateral contraction of the lips and chin; particularly helpful when it appears early in frontal-mesial seizures.

Dialeptic seizure

A seizure whose main manifestation is impaired awareness or unresponsiveness; useful descriptively but not a strong localizer by itself.

Dystonic posturing

Sustained abnormal limb posture, often a powerful lateralizing sign in temporal lobe epilepsy when unilateral.

Epileptogenic zone

The minimum cortical region that must be treated or disconnected to render the patient seizure free; broader than the symptomatogenic zone in many cases.

Figure-of-four sign

Asymmetric tonic posture before or during generalization in which one arm is extended and the other flexed; the extended arm usually points contralateral to seizure onset.

Hypermotor seizure

A seizure dominated by large proximal or axial complex movements such as thrashing, rocking, pedaling, or semipurposeful motor behavior.

Jacksonian march

A gradual spread of clonic or sensory symptoms along the somatotopic map, strongly suggesting sequential recruitment of perirolandic cortex.

Semiology

The clinically observed and experienced manifestations of a seizure, including subjective symptoms, objective signs, behavior, and postictal findings.

Seizure onset zone

The cortical region where the seizure begins on electroclinical analysis; not always identical to the epileptogenic zone.

Symptomatogenic zone

The cortical region whose activation or dysfunction generates a symptom or sign; often close to but not identical with the seizure onset zone.

Temporal-plus epilepsy

A seizure network involving the temporal lobe together with adjacent extratemporal cortex such as temporo-occipital, insular, orbitofrontal, or parietal/perisylvian regions.

Version

Forced, sustained, unnatural turning of the head and eyes to one side, classically lateralizing contralaterally when it is true ictal version.

Index

Entries refer to chapter numbers, section numbers, or appendices rather than dynamic page numbers.

A

B

C

D

E

F

G

H

I

J

K

L

M

N

O

P

R

S

T

V

www.ingramcontent.com/pod-product-compliance
Lightning Source LLC
LaVergne TN
LVHW070954210926
848482LV00002B/215